What'
Alternative?

* ❉ *

Hazel Courteney

WITH DR JOHN BRIFFA

B❉XTREE

C000031296

ADVICE TO THE READER

Before following any medical or dietary advice contained in this book, it is recommended that you consult your doctor if you suffer from any health problems or special conditions or are in any doubt as to its suitability.

First published 1996 by Boxtree, an imprint of
Macmillan Publishers Ltd, 25 Eccleston Place,
London SW1W 9NF and Basingstoke

Associated companies throughout the world

ISBN 0 7522 0514 5

Copyright © Hazel Courteney 1996

The right of Hazel Courteney to be identified as the author
of this work has been asserted by her in accordance with
the Copyright, Designs and Patents Act 1988

All rights reserved. No part of this publication may be reproduced,
stored in or introduced into a retrieval system, or transmitted, in any
form, or by any means (electronic, mechanical, photocopying, recording
or otherwise) without the prior written permission of the publisher.
Any person who does any unauthorized act in relation
to this publication may be liable to criminal prosecution
and civil claims for damages.

1 3 5 7 9 10 8 6 4 2

A CIP catalogue entry for this book is available from the British Library

Typeset by SX Composing DTP, Rayleigh, Essex
Printed in Great Britain by The Bath Press, Bath
Designed by Roger Lightfoot

This book is sold subject to the condition that it shall not, by way of
trade or otherwise, be lent, resold, hired out ot otherwise circulated
without the publisher's prior consent in any form of binding or cover
other than that in which it is published and without a similar condition
including this condition being imposed upon a subsequent purchaser.

I dedicate this book to all people who are searching for optimum health.
Also to those who lost their fight but never stopped trying – for my friend Ralph Marsden who was given another twelve happy years of life thanks to his wife Kathryn's nutritional advice.

For Ralph and Kathryn.

Since my column began in March 1994 I have received hundreds of thank you letters. Here are three of them:

After suffering from a prolonged attack of thrush, I honestly believed there was no cure as my doctor had tried everything. I felt as though I had the plague. After taking the supplements you suggested for just one month, my symptoms completely disappeared. Hazel, I cannot thank you enough, the relief is wonderful and you have given me a new lease of life.

Mrs Caroline Ware, Wimborne, Dorset.

I find your information very interesting and encouraging for so many problems and would like to thank you for providing book titles, telephone numbers and vitamin advice. This has saved me months of visits to health stores and book shops, and a lot of money, as I was pointed in the right direction so quickly. For years I suffered from irritable bowel and psoriasis, but nowadays thanks to your advice I am altogether healthier and feel great.

Mrs Evelyn Empson, Woodbridge, Suffolk.

After taking three courses of antibiotics for a severe sore throat, my doctor felt that he had failed me. Within a few hours of finishing the antibiotics the razor-like throat would return. I honestly thought that taking the vitamins would be a waste of time – but after following your advice for six weeks, not only did my throat problem clear but I felt better than I had in years. I am now taking regular supplements and intend to do so for the foreseeable future.

Mrs Hazel Potter, Liverpool.

Acknowledgements

First and foremost I would like to thank my co-author, nutritional physician and friend Dr John Briffa who really cares.

My personal assistant Lindsey Ross-Jarrett who has the patience of a saint and has spent countless hours sifting through hundreds of research papers to help us bring this book together. Thanks Lindsey – you are a star.

I would like to sincerely thank all the dedicated practitioners who have given so much of their time and energy helping with my research during the past five years. Especially Dr John Stirling, Patrick Holford, Gareth Zeal, Rhaya Jordan, Celia Wright, Angela Dowden, Bob Jacobs and Rohit Mehta. To all the alternative practitioners I have met on my journey who are all so kind and truly caring. Keep up your great work which is urgently needed.

For Marianne and Walter for being so dedicated.

Love and thanks to my brother Bob – for his support and energy.

Last but not least to my husband Stuart and daughter Victoria who have stood by me through thick and thin. Thank you for trusting in me and for being my best friends.

Contents

Why I Wrote this Book

After answering 30,000 readers' letters and having spent almost five years studying the work of the world's top research scientists, nutritional doctors and health professionals, it is crystal clear to me that as much as 90% of all chronic conditions could be prevented. Also, there is a staggering amount of evidence proving that many illnesses can be significantly helped through nutrition and natural means.

We could all live happier, healthier, more productive lives, eventually dying of old age, instead of experiencing a gradual deterioration in health which often ruins the quality of life in our latter years. So many people are led to believe that their ailments are due to their age and resign themselves to a life of ill health and suffering. The truth is that there is so much we could do for ourselves as long as we make the decision to take more responsibility for our own health.

Advances in orthodox medicine have had little or no impact in stemming the tidal wave of chronic illnesses such as heart disease, high blood pressure, cancer and arthritis. In addition, we are now seeing entirely new problems emerge like hyperactivity and aggression in children and lowered sperm counts in men. Incidences of asthma, eczema, cancer and allergies are increasing alarmingly. To understand why there is such an explosion of illness today read the next chapter 'Why You Need Nutritional Supplements'.

After answering so many letters from my column in the *Daily Mail*, I realized there was a desperate need for people to be given information they could trust in an easy-to-read format. After all, most bookshops are packed with health books – surely the public did not need another one? When there is such an enormous amount of information available to us all about health and well-being in magazines, newspapers and on TV programmes, why do so many people continue to be ignorant of the evidence, resulting in an ever-increasing spiral of deteriorating health? Could it be that we simply do not know which information is correct and therefore feel confused as to which way to turn for the truth?

The format of my column proved so useful that I was inundated with letters asking me to write a book of my health hints. Initially, I was appalled that there was any need for me to write a book at all, but I now know with every fibre of my being that this book is urgently needed, as people today are searching for health tips they can trust.

On many occasions I have interviewed people who complain about the lack of information relating to their condition that is being made available to them from their doctor or local clinic. A great majority are truly shocked when I suggest that they are capable of finding alternative therapies and medicines to aid their recovery. I am a firm believer in the body's ability to heal itself; all it needs is the right tools for the job. Every year, the body is renewed to the tune of 98%: your liver is replaced once or twice a year; you have a brand new skeleton every year; your gut lining is completely replaced every 72 hours. As the body is made up from food molecules – your body today is almost entirely made up of what you have eaten during the past year.

Alternatives do work for millions of people – but often doctors have little or no knowledge of alternative medicines and therapies. To be fair, many doctors are stretched to the limit, often working an exhausting schedule under tremendous pressure. Even if this were not the case, there remains the fact that in the course of five years of medical studies, doctors generally receive little or no nutritional training. I have even met a young doctor who said that when she left medical school she did not know whether chicken was mainly protein or starch! So how can we expect our family doctor to know much about vitamins, minerals, herbs, homeopathy or any other alternative treatments? They have enough trouble keeping pace with the constant flow of information in the medical journals about new orthodox treatments. Also new product information is continually being sent to doctors by the pharmaceutical companies, who are all too eager to increase their market share in the lucrative prescription drug market.

Thankfully, the winds of change are beginning to blow in a more positive direction. I have met a few orthodox doctors who suggest supplements and dietary changes instead of prescription drugs in certain cases, often because their own patients are demanding a change. Here and there, conventionally trained doctors such as my co-author are using diet and nutritional supplements exclusively in the treatment of their patients. Some people are actually asking their doctor questions about the side-effects of drugs and are suggesting natural remedies which they have dis-covered are beneficial to their health. People everywhere are sick of being sick and are desperate to find alternatives.

In certain medical practices around the UK you may be lucky enough to find osteopaths, homeopaths, counsellors, nutritionists and occasionally even healers. Increasingly, more and more local health authorities are offering alter-native therapies on the National Health. In fact, some doctors now openly admit that conventional medicine and alternative therapies can work in tandem for the well-being of their patients, whilst many others are still closed to the concept of holistic health.

I have met, interviewed and received thousands of letters from people who have succeeded in changing their habits and discovered alternative ways of healing themselves. Some had eczema or psoriasis, others had heart disorders or arthritis; there were cases involving chronic fatigue syndrome and depression; while many more had suffered and survived life-threatening illnesses like cancer. Now, thanks entirely to sheer determination in their search for answers, most of these people are well.

One dear lady of 83 had suffered from ringing in her ears for nearly 40 years. A friend recommended acupuncture. The therapist suggested vitamins, dietary changes and a short course of acupuncture. The ringing stopped within one month and this wonderful lady is thrilled to have been able to help herself, which has given her renewed self-confidence. Remember, it's never too late! I could recite thousands of stories like this.

Many people discovered alternative therapies through friends, some by investigating and inquiring about the specifics of their condition, others by having their interest awakened by an article they happened to read in a newspaper or magazine. Ultimately, they were all willing to try something new, and over time, many were able to wean themselves off prescription drugs, often with the approval of their doctors. I believe that in the near future a comprehensive service to the patient, in which both alternative and conventional treatments are integrated, will be provided for the benefit of us all. We all urgently need to start practising the art of prevention, as many of us tend to take our bodies for granted until they go wrong.

I am not opposed to conventional medicine, and would not advocate the abolition of prescription drugs, many of which are invaluable for saving lives. Yet so many doctors and pharmaceutical companies dismiss out of hand any and all alternative therapies. Although it is wise to view any new form of treatment with a healthy scepticism, the same goes for any treatment suggested by a doctor, who may be more inclined to prescribe drugs to deal with the symptoms than to look for the root cause of an illness.

No one knows all the answers, but I have been fortunate enough to discover some helpful hints that I know are worth sharing. I have taken great care to outline specific treatments for specific ailments; which supplements to take and where to buy them, in order to make the process as easy as possible. My sole purpose is to help as many people as possible to benefit from the knowledge of my experience. The path you choose to pursue is yours, I merely want to help you find your way.

You can improve the condition of your health and well-being, beginning today. If you are suffering from ill-health, you can begin to turn that around. If you are fortunate enough to enjoy good health, you can make it even better. I say this with confidence even though I don't know you. I hope you will find some useful answers in this book. I have done my best to include most of the advice and remedies which have come my way and which have proved to be beneficial in practice.

The inspiration for this book came from all the wonderful and thought-provoking letters which have been sent to me by the readers of my column. To all of you out there who are suffering from ill health, never give up, the answers are out there. I wish you luck on your road to recovery.

Why You Need Nutritional Supplements

The question I am most often asked when I appear on TV and radio is 'If I eat a sensible diet surely I will get all the vitamins and minerals I need to keep me healthy?'.

In fact, the truth is that as little as 3% of the population in the Western world eat a truly healthy balanced diet. The majority of us talk about healthy eating, but the reality is that we continue to eat far too much junk. In addition, the great majority of us have no idea what actually constitutes a healthy diet. For instance, I have spoken with hundreds of people who believe that consuming numerous cupfuls of tea and coffee is as healthy as drinking plenty of water. They also have no idea that many fizzy drinks are packed with artificial additives and up to eight teaspoonfuls of sugar are added to each can. Recently, a business executive was astounded when I told him that sugar is fattening. It's petrifying what people believe and how much mis-information there is out there.

Eating habits for many of us have changed drastically during recent years. As little as 50 years ago it was routine for the family to sit and eat home-cooked meals with freshly picked vegetables and fruits from a local farm or allotment. Today, this tradition seems to have all but disappeared. Many fruits and vegetables that were once grown locally, are often transported thousands of miles to reach our tables. Once picked, fruits and vegetables can lose up to 50% of their vitamin content in just ten days. Storing fruits and vegetables in the home and the cooking process causes further loss of any remaining nutrients. Tests today also show that at the time of picking, our vegetables and fruits contain approximately 50% less vitamin and mineral content than they did 50 years ago. Why is this?

Since the 1950s fruit and vegetables have been grown using herbicides and pesticides which leach minerals from the soil. Intensive agricultural farming has reduced vital mineral levels. In addition, sulphur from acid rain destroys vital minerals in the soil such as selenium, which is known to help protect against heart disease. In Bulgaria, where the soil is rich in selenium, there is a low incidence of heart disease. In Finland and Denmark, selenium is added to the soil in an effort to correct potential deficiencies.

Not only is our food depleted of vital nutrients, it also contains many unnatural poisons. Over 3,500 chemical preservatives and additives are added to our food, and more than 3,000 toxic substances are in the air we breathe. Figures show that every year, each and every one of us, unless we live on a strictly organic diet – has up to a gallon of pesticides and herbicides sprayed on our fruit and vegetables and almost all of us eat 12lb of food additives! In 1994 a survey of carrots found some to have levels 25 times higher than the safety limit of organophosphates (OPs) and in 1995, 10% of lettuce had excessive pesticide residues. So widespread is the use of these chemicals, they are now finding their way into our water supply. Current estimates are that over 14 million people in the UK consume water with pesticide levels above the permissible limit. Our bodies were not designed to cope with these toxins and we are now reaping a bitter harvest. One in ten of us will have mental health problems, one in three of us will develop cancer and almost half of us will die of either a heart attack or stroke. Why?

Many of us live fast-paced lives, eat in a hurry and often cannot be bothered to cook fresh foods. Instead we tend to rely on processed and pre-packaged foods. Children and many adults love junk, fried and processed foods and sweets, and nearly always choose unhealthy food and drinks even when offered healthy alternatives. In 1995 the British public consumed 10 billion litres of fizzy, caffeinated drinks plus equivalent amounts of tea, coffee and beer. Almost all this refined, pre-packaged and processed food contains virtually no vitamins, minerals or fibre. We are bombarded with food advertisements claiming that products are 'packed with added vitamins'. Have you ever asked yourself *why* they need to add vitamins, if the food is nutritious in the first place?

Dr Richard Passwater, who has been a research scientist for over thirty-five years, states that refined sugar has had 99.9% of all its natural nutrients removed, and the only reason that there is 0.1% nutritional value left is because the sugar companies cannot figure out how to remove the last 0.1%. White flour and mass-produced oils are the same. Tinned foods are sterilized at high temperatures, once canned, to kill any bacteria. How many nutrients do you think are left after these processes?

Many governments suggest minimum amounts of nutrients, called recommended daily allowances (RDAs). In Europe there are RDAs for 13 nutrients and yet there are about 50 essential nutrients required for health. Confusion is rife as RDAs vary from country to country, so who do we believe? The RDAs are designed to prevent obvious signs of deficiency such as scurvy (vitamin C deficiency). However, they do not represent the quantities of nutrients we require for optimum health. Nor do they represent the levels of vitamins and minerals we need to protect our bodies from the pollutants and toxins in our environment. What is more, RDAs take no account of individual requirements such as age, gender or health status of the person.

Some people would like to see new laws passed stating that any formulation containing nutrients over one and a half times the suggested RDA should be classified as a prescription-only medicine. In France, a court judgement early in 1996, ruled that no retail outlet in France could sell supplements containing more than 150mg of vitamin C. Anything over this trifling amount will now require a prescription and will only be available from pharmacies. This is scandalous. I personally take at least 1g (1000mg) of vitamin C each day, but the current RDA is only 60mg. I would have to eat approximately 14 oranges to ingest 1g of vitamin C and it is now widely acknowledged that 60mg is only just enough to prevent scurvy but not enough for optimum health.

It was discovered in the mid-eighteenth century that the consumption of lemons or limes prevented the condition of scurvy. Yet, it took almost 50 years before the British Admiralty finally decided that sailors should be given lemons or limes on every voyage.

Dr Abram Hoffer, a world authority on depression and schizophrenia who has worked in the field of nutritional therapy for nearly 45 years, stated recently that tests carried out in Cambridge have shown that heart attack patients are 75% less likely to have another attack if they include 400iu (international units) of natural vitamin E in their diets. To eat 400iu of vitamin E, you would have to eat around 40 avocados every day! He went on to say that in 1945 in Ontario, Canada, 30,000 people were involved in tests regarding vitamin E with the same results as we have in 1996. Are we going to wait another fifty years before we take any notice, when the proof is readily available for all to see?

I have spent the last five years reading research papers from doctors, research scientists and nutritionists in addition to hundreds of case studies and dozens of books about nutrition. This information is not new, much of it has been around for over 30 years. Without any doubt, we are no longer getting enough vitamins and minerals from our diet for optimum health.

Even though vitamins and minerals come in capsule or tablet form, they are *not* to be confused with prescription medications. We need them to survive and as we cannot manufacture them inside our bodies, we *must* take them in from our diet. Many people ask me, if they take enough vitamins and minerals can they continue eating junk food? I'm afraid the answer is no. Nutritional supplements are a supplement to, not a replacement for a healthy diet.

We all need to start eating food that is as unprocessed and unrefined as possible. Natural organic food, without pesticides and additives, is the way forward. As we near the end of the millennium we need to return to the type of foods that we ate when this century began. But we also need extra help. This is now proven – we *need* to start taking vitamins and minerals to prevent and treat many illnesses.

Important Hints You Need to Know about Supplements

Before reading the hints section, here are a few tips on how best to use your supplements for optimum benefits.

- Supplements taken regularly in the long term almost always produce beneficial effects, but don't expect miracles in a week. Supplements are not magic bullets, but stimulate the body's natural healing processes giving long-term health benefits.
- Generally speaking, supplementation with nutrients produces improvements in health more slowly than prescription medications, which normally just suppress symptoms. If you start a course of vitamins, minerals or any supplements, take them regularly for at least two months in order to see the benefits. Any changes in your health may be very subtle.
- Supplements are known to help prevent many chronic diseases like heart disease and cancer. Here, no apparent benefits may be seen as the additional nutrients suggested provide a form of health insurance.
- Many supplements currently on the market have less than optimum quantities of beneficial ingredients. In general you get what you pay for. Some low-priced supplements contain relatively small amounts of nutrients or forms of nutrients which the body finds difficult to use. The better quality and usually more expensive supplements generally provide better value for money in the long run.

11

- Most vitamins have a good shelf life but will cease to be effective if you keep them for too long. Be aware of sell-by dates and always keep your vitamins in a cool, dry place – never expose them to direct sunlight.
- Supplements should be taken with food unless otherwise stated on the label. This ensures a much better absorption.
- Avoid taking any supplements with tea, coffee or alcohol as these can block absorption of certain nutrients.
- Some people have reactions to certain supplements but this is quite an uncommon occurrence. This is usually caused not by the nutrients themselves but by a reaction to one or more of the other ingredients contained in the supplement. In general, better quality supplements containing hypo-allergenic ingredients are less likely to give rise to adverse reactions. If you suffer a reaction to any supplement, stop taking it immediately.
- Zinc supplements are better absorbed if taken on their own with water in the early evening and it can take 4–6 weeks before zinc becomes operational within the body.
- The supplements suggested in this book can be taken by anyone over the age of 16. For children's dosages, seek professional guidance.
- Probiotics (or friendly bacteria) more commonly known as acidopholis should also contain bifidus strain bacteria. All probiotic preparations keep better in glass bottles and must be kept either in a fridge or freezer.
- If you are pregnant, or planning a pregnancy, do not take any supplement which contains more than 5000iu of vitamin A. Most manufacturers state whether supplements are unsuitable during pregnancy.
- Keep all supplements away from young children. Any substance taken in excess can cause harm. Follow the manufacturer's instructions unless we have stated otherwise.
- *If you are in any doubt about the amount of supplements you or your children should be taking – always consult a qualified health practitioner.*

The Codes – How to Use this Book

Throughout this book I have used codes to identify specific brands. The codes are at the end of each of the sections entitled SUPPLEMENTS. If no code or other details are mentioned, then the listed supplements should be readily available from good health food stores.

No-one is more aware than myself of the hundreds of alternative supplements now available. In this book I have suggested many specific brands which I have used regularly for some years. If I tried to mention every brand by name, this book would not be an easy-to-read book of hints, but a lengthy encyclopaedia. My personal preference for specific brands in no way infers that they are better or more beneficial than others on the market. If you have specific brands you know and trust, check with your own suppliers or health shop who, I am sure, will stock similar supplements to those recommended in the hints section.

BC
BioCare Ltd, Lakeside, Lifford Lane, Kings Norton, Birmingham B30 3NT. Tel: 0121 433 3727 Fax: 0121 433 3879 EMail: 100574,1017@compuserve.com

In America BioCare products are available from: Interplexus INC, 6620 South, 192 Second Place, J-105 Kent, WA98032, USA. Tel: 00 1 206 251 0596

BLK
The House of Blackmores, 37 Rothschild Road, London W4 5HT. Tel: 0181 987 8640 Fax: 0181 987 8641

In Australia; Blackmores, PO Box 258, Balgowlan, NSW 2093, Australia Tel: 00 612 9951 0111

FSC
The Health and Diet Company, Europa Park, Stone Clough Road, Radcliffe, Manchester M26 1GG. Tel: 01204 707420 Fax: 01204 792238. EMail: 101577,1325

HN
Higher Nature Ltd, The Nutrition Centre, Burwash Common, East Sussex TN19 7LX. Tel: 01435 882880 Fax: 01435 883720 EMail: 106004.3606@compuserve.com

LGF
Larkhall Green Farm, 225, Putney Bridge Road, London SW15 2PY. Tel: 0181 874 1130 Fax: 0181 871 0066

NC
The NutriCentre, The Hale Clinic, 7 Park Crescent, London N1N 3HE. Tel: 0171 436 5122 Fax: 0171 436 5171

PN
PharmaNord (UK) Ltd, Spital Hall, Mitford Morpeth, NE61 3PN. Tel: 01670 519989 Fax: 01670 513222

Q
Quest Vitamins, 8 Venture Way, Aston Science Park, Birmingham B7 4AP. Tel: 0121 359 0056 Fax: 0121 359 0313 EMail : info@questvitamins.co.uk

S
Solgar vitamins are available world-wide. To find out

details of your nearest stockist contact the following addresses:

Solgar Vitamins Ltd, Solgar House, Chiltern Commerce Centre, Ashridge Road, Chesham, Buckinghamshire HP5 2PY. Tel: 01494 791691 Fax: 01494 792792

Solgar Vitamin and Herb Company, 500 Willow Tree Road, Leonia, New Jersey 07605 USA. Tel: 00 1 201 944 2311 Fax: 001 201 944 7351

All these companies are happy to post world-wide.

For all other addresses and details, see the Index of Useful Information and Addresses on page 257

Author's Note

In this book I have, in certain instances, suggested specific doses of nutrients. This is usually to ensure that enough of a nutrient is taken to be of benefit in a specific condition. In places where no specific doses have been suggested, take the supplements daily, according to instructions on the label.

This book is not intended as a substitute for conventional medical counselling. Never stop taking prescribed medicine without first consulting your doctor. In matters that pertain to your health, always see your doctor.

ACID STOMACH (*see also* Indigestion and Low Stomach Acid)

During an average lifetime more than 100 tons of food passes through the gut and 300 litres of digestive juices are produced by the body to break it down; it's no wonder that so many of us end up with stomach acidity, indigestion and heartburn. The stomach secretes acid to digest protein, but when the stomach makes too much acid, symptoms such as a burning sensation under the ribs and heartburn may result. This condition can be caused by stress, exhaustion, eating the wrong foods together and heavy, rich meals. (Never underestimate how prolonged stress and exhaustion can seriously affect your digestive system and your overall health.)

Diet

Many of us eat or drink too many acid-forming foods such as coffee, tea, alcohol, spicy foods, sugar, cakes, biscuits, meat, dairy products, orange juice, chocolate and artificial sweeteners. Eliminating or reducing these foods can significantly decrease symptoms. Eat more foods which tend to alkalize the body like fresh fruits, vegetables and sprouts. Raw vegetables contain enzymes which aid digestion, therefore buy a vegetable juicer and blend any mixture of fresh fruits and vegetables. My favourite is apple, carrot, celery, broccoli and root ginger. Drink immediately after juicing whilst all the enzymes and vitamins are still alive. Reduce alcohol and stop smoking: these can both aggravate an acid stomach.

Supplements

Sea Plasma (a concentrated source of natural beta carotene derived from sea plankton) helps to alkalize the system. Take with each meal or try spirulina or chlorella which are also sea algae products. Citrase (containing calcium and magnesium) alkalizes and calms an acid stomach.

Gastroplex, a supplement containing slippery elm, marsh-mallow and gamma oryzanol, soothes the lining of the stomach. • [BC]

Reading
The Food Combiner's Meal Planner by Kathryn Marsden, £4.99, Thorsons. A valuable handbook telling you which foods are acid- and alkaline-forming.
Food Combining in 30 Days by Kathryn Marsden, £4.99, Thorsons.
Stomach Ulcers and Acidity by Dr Leonard Mervyn, £2.99, Thorsons.

Hints
Anything which makes digestion easier will help ease an acid stomach. Chew all foods thoroughly and avoid drinking too much with meals, as this dilutes the secretions responsible for digestion. Eat little and often, avoiding large, heavy meals. The larger the meal, the greater the burden on the stomach, causing further discomfort. Small meals are especially important if you are stressed, as stress may increase stomach acid and impair digestion. Ensure meal times are as unhurried as possible. Never eat large meals when upset. If you are prone to nervous conditions, join a yoga class and learn to relax. Get plenty of exercise but do not exercise immediately after eating.

Food combining helps an acid stomach: this means separating proteins and starches to aid digestion; basically if you are eating a protein like meat or fish, eat this with salad or vegetables but not potatoes, pasta or bread; conversely when you eat bread, pasta or potatoes, eat them with vegetables or salad, not protein. Many people become reliant on antacids to control their symptoms, when making a few simple changes to the diet and eating pattern can produce very significant relief in the majority of cases. Antacids can harm the body if used excessively and many contain large amounts of aluminium which has been implicated in Alzheimer's disease; others contain magnesium which, when taken in excess, can cause clumsiness, drowsiness and confusion.

ACNE

Acne is common in adolescence and is caused by blockages in the skin's sebaceous glands. These make an oily substance called sebum which is used to lubricate the skin. In adolescence, hormonal changes are often a major factor in the development of acne. In adulthood, spots and acne often result from internal toxicity in the body which can be caused by a variety of factors including constipation, bacterial or yeast overgrowth **(see Candida)** or a food sensitivity. The liver is mainly responsible for filtering toxins from the system. When the liver becomes overloaded, toxins are dumped by the body into the skin. The key to controlling acne is to reduce toxicity in the body.

Diet

Try eating only fruit and vegetables accompanied by lots of mineral water for three days and then maintain a healthy diet that includes fresh, unprocessed foods such as fruits, vegetables, wholemeal bread, brown rice and pulses. Avoid fatty foods such as red meat, dairy products made from cows' milk, processed foods and greasy take-away meals. Sugar in any form should be avoided including pre-packaged biscuits, cakes and chocolate. Essential fatty acids are vital for healthy skin, therefore include linseeds, sunflower seeds and pumpkin seeds in your everyday diet **(*see* General Health Hints *and* Fats You Need To Eat)**.

Supplements

For six weeks take 15mg of natural beta-carotene plus 3g of vitamin C daily. If you suffer from acne which flares up prior to your period, take 50–100mg of B6 daily plus a B complex. Zinc is vital for skin healing. Take 30–60mg zinc picolinate daily for six weeks along with 200iu vitamin E. • **[FSC]**

Greenfood supplements, such as green wheat grass extracts, chlorella, blue-green algae and spirulina all act as cleansers and help to alkalize the system. These are available from good health food stores. If you have been taking antibiotics take at least two acidophilus capsules daily for one month to help restore the good bacteria in the gut which some antibiotics can destroy.

Reading

Super Skin by Kathryn Marsden, £5.99, Thorsons.

Hints

To cleanse the skin use Hi Tech Hygiene special soap and facial baths. Also spray colloidal silver (which is a natural antibiotic) onto the affected skin. For details call 01435 882880.

The Sher System is a skin regime especially formulated for problem skin and further details can be obtained from The Sher System, 30 New Bond Street, London W1Y 9HD or call 0171 499 4022.

Rosa Mosqueta, a Latin American plant-based oil, has been used topically to heal acne scars. For details call 0171 436 5122.

Exercise encourages free flow of sebum and de-toxification of the body through sweating. Many readers have benefited from taking aloe vera juice internally and by using the gel externally.

AGEING

Ageing is a natural process, but the rate at which we age is, to a degree, under our control. Many people say you are as old as you feel, and a positive mental outlook coupled with a healthy diet are vital if you want to slow the ageing process. People who are negative and angry tend to age faster than happy, relaxed people. In a recent study in the United States, a group of men in their seventies were installed in a University campus which had been transformed into a replica University from the 1950s. The men were dressed in clothes from the fifties and asked to behave just as they did when attending college. After three weeks the researchers assessed each individual for the biological age by measuring factors such as muscle strength and blood pressure. Incredibly, biological age had decreased by an average of three years! Start thinking young – it really does help.

Ageing is largely due to the effect of damaging substances in the body called 'free radicals'. Free radicals are dangerous chemicals which are produced continuously in the body. Their production is increased through inhaling cigarette smoke, car exhaust fumes, pollution and by eating fried, barbecued or fatty food. Excessive alcohol, stress and over-exposure to sunlight also increase free radical damage. Whilst you cannot completely avoid free radicals you can protect yourself, by making sure your diet is rich in antioxidant nutrients such as vitamins A, C and E, natural carotenes like beta carotene and lycopene, and the mineral selenium, which as scientists have proved, can neutralize free radicals.

Diet

There is little point in taking vitamins and supplements to combat the ageing process if your diet is unhealthy. Drink at least one litre of filtered or bottled water daily. Eat plenty of brown rice, brown bread, lentils, beans, organic vegetables, fruits, nuts and seeds. Eating too much refined sugar speeds up the ageing process and depletes the body of chromium, potassium, magnesium and zinc. Avoid saturated fats found mainly in red meat, dairy produce and all junk foods which can block the pores in the skin and also accelerate ageing. For beautiful skin we need essential fatty acids. These are found in linseeds, sunflower seeds and pumpkin seeds (*see* **General Health Hints** *and* **Fats You Need To Eat**).

Supplements
Daily regime for women: 2g of vitamin C as magnesium ascorbate plus one B complex which are essential for the nervous system, skin, nail and hair health. NutriGuard Forte containing natural carotenes, vitamins A, C, E and selenium and a new high potency antioxidant called lycopene. Zinc ascorbate helps to support the immune system. Women over forty should also take a multi-vitamin/mineral like Femforte which is designed especially for women. CoQ10 Plus (containing Co-Enzyme Q10, flaxseed oil, vitamin E and lecithin), aids energy production, helps protect the heart, aids circulation, protects the skin and supports the immune system. • **[BC]**

For beautiful skin (and a healthier brain and digestive system), we need to take essential fatty acids daily. EFAs are found in organic, unrefined linseed, pumpkin and sunflower oils and seeds. To save me eating seeds all day, I take Essential Balance Oil (*for further details see* **Fats You Need To Eat**).

Daily regime for men: 1g of vitamin C plus zinc ascorbate to help protect the prostate from disease and maintain the sperm count. In addition, NutriGuard Forte, (see above), 300iu of vitamin E to help reduce free radical damage and reduce the risk of heart disease. A multi-vitamin and mineral complex. • **[BC]**

(*Also see* **Fats You Need To Eat**.)

Reading
Ageless Body, Timeless Mind by Deepak Chopra, £7.99, Rider.
Optimum Nutrition by Patrick Holford, £5.95, ION Press.
Stop Ageing Now by Jean Carper, £9.99, Thorsons.
The New Super Nutrition by Dr Richard Passwater, £5.99,
Pocket Books. To order call 0171 436 5122.
New Anti-Ageing by Leslie Kenton, £6.99, Vermillion.

Hints
Get plenty of exercise but not to excess. Meditation reduces
stress which can age us faster than any other condition (*see*
Meditation). Too much sun is ageing but we do need some
sunshine to produce vitamin D, which helps to keep bones
healthy. Wear a sunscreen during the summer months whenever you are outside to protect the skin. As moisture is so vital
to ageing skin, invest in a humidifier and use it in the bedroom.

Laser therapy can help remove the visible signs of ageing,
like liver spots. For further details contact Laser Care, 1 Park
View, Harrogate, North Yorkshire HG1 5LY. Tel: 01423
563827.

ALCOHOL
Moderate consumption of alcohol is associated with a
reduced risk of heart disease. The health benefits of alcohol
seem to be clearer in men than in women, where an increase
in certain cancers, for example cancer of the breast, seem to
outweigh other benefits. On a dietary level, there is not
much to recommend about alcohol. The nutrient content is
low, but high in calories. Alcohol irritates the lining of the
gut which plays an important part in the development of
food sensitivities (*see* **Allergies**). Alcohol has a direct toxic
affect on the liver thereby reducing this organ's ability to

filter toxins from the blood.

Diet

Eat plenty of fruit and vegetables, or consume fresh fruit and vegetable juices, especially those containing beetroot which is very cleansing. Fresh raw vegetables, especially broccoli, cabbage, cauliflower and artichokes contain chemicals which help the liver detoxify more efficiently. Drink a glass of mineral or filtered water for every alcoholic drink you consume to help prevent dehydration and allow the body to detoxify more efficiently. Hangovers are the result of dehydration, toxicity and low blood sugar. If you suffer a hangover, a freshly made fruit or vegetable juice with a banana will help to re-hydrate the body as well as restoring blood sugar levels. Avoid coffee and tea which further dehydrate the body.

Supplements

The herb milk thistle is known to help with liver function and cleansing. As alcohol depletes the body of vital nutrients, take 1g of vitamin C plus one multi-vitamin/mineral high in B vitamins to speed elimination of alcohol from the body. • [LGF]

The herb kudzu which helps inhibit alcohol craving as well as being used in the treatment of alcoholism. • [FSC]

To avoid a hangover either take 1g of linseed oil or 1g of evening primrose oil prior to going to bed. The active ingredient in evening primrose oil, called gamma linolenic acid, is a natural painkiller.

Hints

If you are going to drink then it is wise to spread your drinking out over the course of the week rather than bingeing on one or two days. Better quality red wine seems to confer the most health benefits, due to antioxidant substances called polyphenols, present in the skin of red grapes. The skin of white grapes is discarded during the processing of white wine.

Dandelion tea is excellent for cleansing the liver and kidneys. Remember it takes 20 minutes for alcohol to have an effect and over one hour for the body to process each unit. (One unit = half a pint of beer, a small glass of wine or a single measure of spirits). If you are concerned about the amount that you (or a member of your family) are drinking, call Drinkline, a national alcohol helpline, on 0345 320202 or 0171 332 0202 in London; or their 24-hour recorded information service on 0500 801802. All calls are treated in the strictest confidence and Drinkline provides a full support service for people with drink problems as well as their families.

ALLERGIC RHINITIS (*see also* **Allergies** *and* **Hayfever**)
Symptoms of allergic rhinitis are a runny nose, sneezing, sinus congestion and runny or itchy eyes. This condition is common during the summer months when the high pollen count gives rise to 'hay fever'. If symptoms occur all year round, the trigger is likely to be a food allergy or dust. Animal hair, perfumes, paint and sudden temperature changes are also common triggers.

Diet
This problem is often associated with a sensitivity to cows' milk or milk products although other foods such as chocolate, orange juice or wheat can also be to blame. Keeping a food diary can help identify the culprits. Soya or rice milk are non-dairy, low-fat alternatives to cows' milk products. Many individuals who are sensitive to cows' milk often find they are better able to tolerate goats' or sheeps' milk products.

Supplements

Take two acidophilus capsules daily for one month, to maintain the good bacteria in the gut that is vital for proper digestion. Inadequate digestion can lead to allergic reactions, therefore also take a digestive enzyme capsule regularly with main meals.

Supplements like echinacea, garlic, horseradish and chloride compound help boost the immune system and reduce symptoms when an attack is very severe. Take 3g of vitamin C with bioflavonoids daily, along with 300iu of vitamin E which have a natural anti-histamine effect. • **[BLK]**

Reading

Not all in the Mind by Dr Richard Mackarness, £7.99, Thorsons.
The Allergy Survival Guide by Jane Houtton, £10.99, Vermillion.
Allergies by Stephen Terrass, £4.99, Thorsons.

Hints

During an acute attack, a homeopathic nasal spray called Euphorbium Spray is extremely effective. It helps to relieve a runny nose, congestion and headaches. • **[NC]**

Dust and other airborne allergens can be reduced in your immediate environment with an ioniser.

Try New Era tissue salts for allergic rhinitis – from any good pharmacy or health food store.

A course of Hi Tech Hygiene facial baths will cleanse the nasal passages and sinuses. For details call 01435 882880.

ALLERGIES

Increasing numbers of people are suffering from allergies due to any number of potential triggers including food, chemicals, pollution, cigarette smoke and pollen. The body has a limited capacity to cope with potential allergens and when this limit is exceeded, symptoms start to appear. This is why it is possible to develop problems like hay fever and food sensitivity at any age. There are now over 3,500 food additives in use and an average person ingests 4.5kg of these a year, ten times the amount we ate thirty years ago. A further 3,000 chemicals such as lead and cadmium are in our polluted air. Our bodies are not designed to deal with this quantity of chemicals and for those who suffer allergies, the body is simply saying that it has had enough.

Diet
Many food sensitivities have their basis in a leaky gut, where undigested foods leak through the gut wall causing an aller-gic response. Improving digestion and eating the right diet can be of enormous benefit in reducing allergic reactions (*see* **Acid Stomach** *for tips on digestion*). Eat a natural wholefood diet (*see* **General Health Hints**), whilst avoiding totally for at least two months any foods to which you know you are sen-sitive. The commonest culprits are wheat, dairy produce, yeast, eggs and oranges. It is often the foods you crave the most that are causing the problem! Most cravings take about a month to break so be patient with yourself.

Supplements
Histazyme, a complex containing calcium, vitamin C, zinc, bromelain, silica, vitamin A and manganese which acts as a natural anti-histamine. HEP194 containing the herb silymarin, the enzyme lipase, the amino acid methionine and B vitamins which help cleanse the liver. Two acidophilus capsules daily for six weeks to replace the good bacteria in the gut and aid digestion

A multi-vitamin plus 3g of vitamin C daily. Two GLA capsules (gamma linolenic acid, an essential fatty acid) to help heal the leaky gut. • **[BC]**

The amino acid glutamine helps to heal the gut and reduce allergic responses, especially when a food allergy is suspected. Take with each meal. Aloe vera juice can help reduce allergic tendencies. Take three tablespoons daily in juice or water. • [HN]

Reading
The Allergy Survival Guide by Jane Houtton, £10.99, Vermilion.
Not All In The Mind by Dr Richard Mackarness, £7.99, Thorsons.
Food Allergy and Nutrition Revolution by Dr James Braly, £16.15, Keats Publishing. Available to order from 0171 436 5122.
Allergies by Stephen Terrass, £4.99, Thorsons.
Poisons Around Us by Hennry A Schroeder, £10.99, Keats.

Hints
Fresh cabbage juice is high in L Glutamine, known to help to heal a leaky gut. Cover one pound of organic cabbage with filtered water, bring to the boil and simmer for twenty minutes. Strain and sip the cooled liquid.

Many allergic and chemically sensitive people can benefit enormously by switching from tap water to mineral or filtered water instead. Tests in America found that 98% of environmentally ill patients improved just by eliminating tap water. An excellent water filter is Watersimple from The Fresh Water Filter Company. For further details contact them at: Carlton House, Aylmer Road, Leytonstone, London E11 3AD or call 0181 558 7495.

There is an allergy blood test called the Immuno Test, £295. A free allergy fact sheet plus details of the allergy test are available by sending a large SAE to Higher Nature, The Nutrition Centre, Burwash Common, East Sussex TN19 7LX.

To test if you have a food allergy, first take your resting

pulse rate. Then eat a food to which you think you may be sensitive, like bread or milk. Wait 15 to 30 minutes and take your pulse again. If your pulse has increased by more than ten beats a minute, it is likely that you have a sensitivity to the test food.

Medivac Vacuum Cleaner is an excellent and effective high powered vacuum which does not give out dust in its exhaust. Further details available on 01625 539401.

Honeywell make a room air filter called Envirocare which removes all known airborne allergens from the room. For details call Essential Systems on 01344 874573.

ALZHEIMER'S DISEASE (*see also* **Memory**)

Alzheimer's disease is a progressive, degenerative disease that attacks the brain, resulting in dementia which is characterised by memory loss – particularly short-term memory – and decreased intellectual functioning. Theories abound as to the cause of this condition, and many scientists believe that aluminium and mercury poisoning are important factors. Recent research suggests that free radicals (*see* **Ageing**) have an important role to play in the development of this condition and that by taking anti-oxidant vitamins and minerals we may well be able to delay or slow down progression of symptoms. Many people who start to lose their memory automatically think they are becoming senile or have Alzheimer's and many scientists now believe that many cases are misdiagnosed. Often, memory loss is caused by decreasing circulation in the brain. By eating the right foods and taking supplements, memory can often be improved (*see also* **Memory**).

Diet

The brain needs certain nutrients to function properly.

Many pollutants found in food and air affect our body's function and ultimately have an adverse affect on the brain. Many elderly people do not eat sufficient quantities of fresh foods – which contain vital vitamins and minerals to feed their brains – nor do they ingest sufficient essential fatty acids (found in linseeds, sunflower and pumpkin seeds and fish) which are vital for brain function. *See* **General Health Hints** *and* **Fats You Need To Eat**.

Supplements

Alzheimer's disease sufferers seem to have a deficiency in the vital brain chemical acetylcholine. This results in poor memory, lethargy, decreased dreaming and a dry mouth. Take one tablespoon of lecithin granules daily on your cereal, but make sure the product you buy contains more than 30% of phosphatidyl choline. Many elderly people lack vitamin B, especially B12, therefore a B complex including B12 should be included. Phosphatidyl Serine extracted from soya beans is known to improve depression associated with dementia, repair damage to nerve centres and, in some cases, to reverse damage within the brain. This is a highly specialized supplement, and a dose of between 300–500mg daily is required. • **[S]**

Brain Food is a supplement developed especially to feed the brain, containing niacin (B3), pantothenic acid (B5), phosphatidyl choline, arginine and DMAE. Take three daily. NADH is a co-enzyme supplement which has proved helpful in some cases by improving mental function. • **[HN]**

Studies have shown that a daily intake of the herb gingko biloba improves the circulation in the brain and may help restore memory and normal behaviour. Take 200mg of standardized extract daily (do not buy cheap gingko extracts).

Take an antioxidant complex, a multi-mineral complex and 200iu of vitamin E to help protect the brain from further free radical damage.

Two GLA (gamma linolenic acid – an essential fatty acid) improves blood supply to the brain. • **[BC]**

Reading
Coping With Alzheimer's – A Care Giver's Emotional Survival Guide by Rose Oliver and Frances Bock, £8.99, Wiltshire Books.
Alzheimer's and Other Confusional States by Dr Gerry Bennett, £5.99, Optima.
Alzheimer's: A Practical Guide For Carers To Help You Through The Day by Frena Gray-Davidson, £8.99, Piatkus Books.

Hints
Certain prescription drugs are known to cause side-effects which appear similar to symptoms of senile dementia. Anyone who feels that they may have the onset of dementia should immediately consult a qualified doctor, who is also a nutritionist (*see* **Useful Information**). In certain cases, the removal of mercury (amalgam dental fillings) has assisted with the recovery of some faculties (*see* **Mercury Fillings**). Because of the link between aluminium and Alzheimer's, avoid aluminium cooking utensils and pans, and food stored in aluminium containers. Many antiperspirants contain aluminium, so use a natural deodorant. Simple antacids are often based on aluminium salts and should also be avoided. Because the food additive monosodium glutamate has recently been linked to Alzheimer's, avoid all foods containing MSG. Many experts state that if our mineral levels are low, then the body tends to absorb more aluminium – hence the importance of taking a multi-mineral daily.

Some people report that homeopathy has improved their condition. See a qualified homeopath who is also a doctor (*see* **Useful Information** *for further details*). The brain needs to be kept working at all costs – there certainly is some truth in the phrase 'use it or lose it' as far as the brain is concerned.

Keep doing crosswords and force the brain to work by counting down from 1,000 each day in multiples of various numbers; such as 1,000 less 7 = 993, less 7 = 986, etc. Many pesticides have been linked to neurological problems and these chemicals are finding their way into our drinking water. Therefore use a good water filter that removes all of these residues.

ANAEMIA

Every part of the body needs oxygen to survive. Oxygen is transported around the body attached to a substance called haemoglobin which is contained in red blood cells. Anaemia occurs if the concentration of haemoglobin drops below a certain level, resulting in symptoms such as fatigue, headaches and faintness.

Several nutrients are essential for the manufacture of haemoglobin. Iron, vitamin B12 and folic acid are the most important and if any of these are deficient in the diet, anaemia can result. Iron deficiency is the most common cause of anaemia and rarely results from a straightforward deficiency in the diet. It is caused by losing more blood than the body can replace naturally. In women, the most common cause of excessive blood loss is heavy periods. Persistent, heavy menstrual bleeding should be investigated by your doctor. Anaemia due to B12 deficiency is quite common in vegans as B12 is not found in any non-animal foods except for sea algae, such as chlorella or spirulina. As anaemia can have many causes, if you think you are anaemic, consult your doctor.

Diet

Iron and folic acid can be found in lean red meat, poultry, liver, eggs, green leafy vegetables, sesame and sunflower seeds and wholegrain bread. Vitamin B12 is found in kidney, liver, egg, herring, mackerel, cheese and seafood. Too much tea, coffee and alcohol inhibit up to 90% of iron absorption from food. Many people over fifty have digestive problems and do not absorb nutrients properly (*see* **General Health Hints**).

Supplements

Vitamins C and B aid absorption of iron – take these vitamins with your iron tablet or take a ready-mixed formula like Spatone or Floradix which already include these vitamins.

The best forms of iron to take are ferrous gluconate or iron amino acid chelate. Iron reduces the amount of zinc in the body, therefore include a multi-mineral supplement containing zinc in your daily regime.

Reading

Optimum Nutrition by Patrick Holford, £5.95, ION Press. To order, call 0181 877 9993.

Hints

Iron is so vital for health that we store it in our bodies, but if taken in excessive amounts, it can become toxic and is known to cause constipation in some cases. No-one should take iron supplements unless blood tests show anaemia or a medical condition that requires iron. The exception to this is women who suffer from heavy periods and are feeling exhausted. Pregnant women can benefit from formulas such as Floradix or Spatone.

As we age our stomach acid levels fall which means that nutrients are often poorly absorbed from the foods we eat. Take a digestive enzyme with meals to improve absorption.

If large amounts of iron are recommended because of anaemia, then it is best to see a qualified nutritionist who can re-balance your diet and supplements (*see* **Useful Information** *for further details*).

There is a genetic disorder called Haemochromatosis, which affects one in every 200 women, in which iron and large amounts of vitamin C should not be taken. A simple blood test can detect this condition.

ANGINA

Angina Pectoris is caused by an inadequate supply of oxygen to the heart muscle and is usually brought on by exertion or stress. Invariably, angina is caused by a narrowing of the coronary arteries which supply blood to the heart. Typical symptoms include a constricting pain in the centre of the chest which may spread to the neck, jaw and/or the left arm. **If you have any of these symptoms, it is imperative to seek medical attention immediately.** The pain of angina is sometimes accompanied by breathlessness, faintness, sweating or nausea.

Diet

If angina has been diagnosed, start by eating a healthier diet. Avoid junk and processed foods which are high in saturated fat and more likely to speed the rate of narrowing of the coronary arteries. Avoid salt at all times, especially in processed and pre-packaged food. Salt is a major risk factor for high blood pressure (which increases risk of heart disease). Eat plenty of oily fish like mackerel, herrings and salmon, which contain omega 3 oils that are known to protect the heart. Use extra virgin olive oil, a mono-unsaturated fat, instead of saturated animal fats and never cook with margarines which contain harmful fats; use Vitaquell or SuperSpread, which are healthier. Never fry your food; steam, boil, roast or grill. Avoid sugar and shop-bought cakes and full cream dairy products like cheese and cream. Use oat, soya or rice milk instead. Eat plenty of fresh fruit, vegetables and wholegrains like brown rice, brown bread and pulses. Add a tablespoon of linseeds, rich in essential fats to your cereal each day. Garlic is known to thin the blood, so use plenty in cooking and eat it in its raw state whenever possible.

Supplements

Bio-Magnesium, as magnesium is known to help regulate heart beat. NutriGuard Forte (containing natural beta-carotene and lycopene, vitamins E, A and C plus the mineral selenium); these are all vital nutrients to assist the heart muscle and aid circulation. Ginkgo Plus, containing bilberry and potassium ascorbate (a form of vitamin C) to strengthen the capillaries and improve circulation. • [BC]

Co-enzyme Q10 is known to protect the heart. A particularly potent formula containing 100mg of CoQ10 is made by Pharma Nord. For details call 0800 591756.

If you are not on blood-thinning drugs, take a garlic capsule regularly.

Vitamin C and the amino acid lysine work together to reverse atherosclerosis, the root of angina. Try Lysine C daily. • [HN]

Reading

The Natural Way With Heart Disease by Richard Thomas, £3.99, Element Books.
Coping With Angina by Louise M Wallace, £7.99, Thorsons.
Super Nutrition for a Healthy Heart by Patrick Holford, £2.50, ION Press.
Eradicating Heart Disease by Matthias Rath MD, £14.20, Health Now. Available to order from 0171 436 5122.

Hints

If you are overweight then it is wise to lose weight. Rather than going on a strict diet, this is best achieved by eating healthily. If you are a smoker, then it is imperative that you stop. With your doctor's permission, embark on a programme of gentle exercise. Start by walking or swimming for 15 minutes daily, gradually building to 30 minutes or more. Yoga is an excellent form of relaxation, which reduces stress and teaches you how to breathe more efficiently.

Watch *Linus Pauling's New Theory of Heart Disease* video, £9.95 from The Institute of Optimum Nutrition, tel: 0181 877 9993. It explains how people have been helped by mega doses of vitamin C and lysine.

ANTIBIOTICS (*see also* **Candida**)

Antibiotics may kill the bacteria causing an infection, but many can also deplete the gut of the healthy bacteria which have an essential role to play in gut and general health. Bacteria can also develop an immunity to antibiotics over time, creating new resistant strains. Antibiotics suppress natural immune function in the long term. This immune dampening effect, along with a loss of healthy bacteria in the gut can allow fungal infections such as candida to flourish. Antibiotics are often prescribed for infections caused by viruses such as colds and flu for which they are completely ineffective. The secret to preventing and fighting infections effectively is to keep our immune system strong and healthy. Nutrition has a vital role to play in this process.

Diet

As meat often contains antibiotic residues, choose organically-reared meat and poultry. Fresh organic fruits and vegetables are packed with immune boosting nutrients. Sugar and junk foods, and drinks containing refined sugar, such as colas and pre-packaged desserts, should be kept to a minimum. High levels of sugar in the blood have been shown to reduce the function of the immune system (*see* **General Health Hints**).

Supplements

If you have been taking antibiotics, take two acidophilus daily for one month to replace the friendly bacteria in the gut or take Replete, a concentrated acidophilus formula for seven days after completing any antibiotic course. Take 3g of vitamin C plus a multi-vitamin and mineral complex to boost the immune system. Whilst infection lasts, take 6 grapefruit seed capsules a day until symptoms are relieved, which acts as a natural alternative to conventional antibiotics. • [BC]

The herb cat's claw tea is a powerful immune booster. Silver has been used for centuries as an antibiotic. Pioneers crossing America in their wagon trains always put a silver dollar in the milk to stop it going off and NASA uses a silver water system for its space shuttle. Colloidal Silver is tasteless and highly effective without any negative side-effects. • [HN]

Reading

Superbug: Nature's Revenge by Geoffrey Cannon, £15.99, Virgin Publishing.

Hints

Bee propolis is a natural antibiotic used by bees to sterilize their hives. Many therapists and doctors find that that two propolis capsules taken every day with at least one gram of vitamin C can lead to a general improvement in health and enhanced resistance to infections. For a brochure on bee propolis, send a SAE to: Bee Health Ltd, The Honey Farm, Race Course Road, East Ayton, Scarborough YO13 9HT.

A naturopath or nutritionist should be able to help you to restore your immune system (*see* **Useful Information** *for further details*).

APHRODISIACS, MALE

There are many potential causes for a man to lose either his desire for sex, or his ability to get (or maintain) an erection. This problem is often related to stress and, by dealing with stress effectively, sexual function can, in many cases, be restored. Excessive alcohol consumption is a common cause of sexual difficulties. Some men find that regular strenuous exercise can lead to a deterioration in sexual function, while others report quite the opposite effect. Smoking is another common trouble spot, because it can reduce the blood flow that is essential for erectile function.

Diet

Make sure your diet is high in organic vegetables and fruits and low in animal fat and salt. Red meat should be replaced by free-range chicken and fish. Caffeine and alcohol intake should be limited, as excessive consumption of either of these can have an adverse effect on libido (*see* **General Health Hints**).

Supplements

There is a supplement especially made for men called Virilactin, which includes vitamins like B and E, and the mineral zinc, which are vital for male glandular activity. Also extracts of oysters, a natural source of zinc, and herbs like kava kava, dong quai and Spanish saffron are all recognized for their aphrodisiac qualities. Try one or two a day, when required. • **[LGF]**

Ginkgo biloba 60–120mg of standardized extract improves micro circulation. • **[FSC]**

Reading

The Complete Book of Men's Health by Dr Sara Brewer, £9.99, Thorsons.

Sex Drive by Donald Norfolk, £5.99, Hodder Headline. Available from Green Library on 0171 385 0012.

Super Potency At Any Age by Dr Edwin Flatto, £7.99, Thorsons.

Hints
Eat plenty of pumpkin seeds, which are high in zinc and believed to have libido-enhancing qualities. The reputed aphrodisiac qualities of oysters are probably explained by their high zinc content. Make sure you get plenty of exercise (but not too strenuous!) and fresh air to aid relaxation. By constantly worrying about your lack of sex drive, you often make the situation worse. Studies show that a lack of vitamins C, E, A, B and the minerals zinc and selenium can cause a low sperm count and lack of sex drive. Anyone taking regular antidepressants or sleeping pills may be lacking in these nutrients. Prolonged use of anabolic steroids or cannabis can also impair sexual function. If the condition continues, or you are worried about infertility as well as impotency, see a doctor who is also a nutritionist (*see* **Useful Information** *for further details*).

ARTHRITIS

Osteo-arthritis
Osteo-arthritis is characterized by progressive degeneration of the cartilage which cushions the joints. There is a tendency for the bones around the joint to become weakened and deformed. Typically, it affects the weight bearing joints such as the hips and knees, the spine and also the hands.

Diet
Arthritis sufferers tend to eat too many acid-forming foods and too much of the wrong types of fats. This theme appears

again and again throughout this book and if many of us in the West were to eat less saturated fat and more alkaline-forming foods like millet, organic fruits and vegetables, then many of the acid condition illnesses would be eradicated. Reduce acid-forming foods such as grains, meat, fish and dairy produce. Tea, coffee, alcohol, colas, sugary drinks, red meat, sausages, refined white flour products, bread, cakes and biscuits are all especially acid-forming and should be kept to a minimum. Eat plenty of fresh fruit salad, especially cherries which are anti-inflammatory, but avoid oranges, rhubarb and plums, which are acidic. Include lots of organic green vegetables especially cabbage, broccoli and kale in your daily diet. Eat plenty of oily fish like salmon and mackerel, and choose free-range poultry in preference to red meat. Use extra virgin olive oil for cooking and salad dressings. Include linseeds in your diet every day as they are packed with essential fats which have an anti-inflammatory effect. If you have a juicer, try the following mix each day to re-alkalize your system: carrot, celery, cabbage and a tiny piece of chopped fresh root ginger, which is highly anti-inflammatory. Drink it straight from the juicer while the enzymes and vitamins are alive.

Supplements

There are so many vitamins and minerals known to help arthritic conditions, I have listed the ones likely to prove most beneficial in order of importance.

Take these supplements for at least three months. Ligazyme plus Colleginase contain vital nutrients like calcium, boron, vitamin C, digestive enzymes, magnesium, rutin, silica, vitamins A and D to support connective tissue and aid healing. Bio-Acidophilus on an empty stomach to replace good bacteria in the gut and aid digestion. Pantothenic acid (vitamin B5) deficiency is often associated with arthritis. • [BC]

Essential fatty acids are vital for producing secretions that lubricate our joints. Take two tablespoons of Essential Balance Oil made from organic linseeds, pumpkin and sunflower seeds every day with your vegetable juice. This oil should never be heated and needs to be kept in the fridge. Reduce to one tablespoon daily after eight weeks. • [HN]

Glucosamine sulphate, an amino sugar, has proved helpful in chronic arthritis, try at least three x 500mg for three weeks, thereafter two daily for eight to twelve weeks, which is particularly useful when mobility is impaired. It needs to be taken for at least nine months to actually repair cartilage. For details ask at your health store or call 0171 436 5122.

Cat's claw is a herb that helps to alkalize the system and is highly anti-inflammatory. Take at least three capsules daily for two months and then have a break for a month before starting again. • [S]

Rheumatoid arthritis – RA
RA is characterized by inflammation in the joints and tissues caused by the immune system reacting to the lining of the joint (the synovium). Usually, the disease is chronic and progressive, but the normal course of events is for pain and stiffness to come and go over time. Rheumatoid arthritis affects three times as many women as men.

Diet
Unlike osteo-arthritis, there is mounting evidence that rheumatoid arthritis is linked to food sensitivities. The common culprits appear to be dairy products made from cows' milk, wheat and members of the nightshade family, such as tomatoes, potatoes, aubergines and red and green peppers (capsicum). There is also an association between RA and foods high in oxalic acid. The main foods to avoid are: tea, coffee, chocolate, peanuts, spinach, rhubarb and beetroot (*see dietary advice for* **Osteo-arthritis**). Add cold organic walnut/sunflower oils to salads. Eat more linseeds

and sunflower, and pumpkin seeds (*see* **General Health Hints**).

Supplements

Boswellic acid complex is highly anti-inflammatory and contains boswellic acid, ginger concentrate, turmeric and bilberry flavonoids. Also OptiZinc and Mega EPA 1,000, containing fish oils, lecithin and vitamin E, all beneficial for RA because of their anti-oxidant and anti-inflammatory effects and increases collagen production. • **[BC]**

A multi-mineral containing calcium, magnesium, boron and selenium to help keep bones healthy. Pantothenic Acid (B5) with a B complex • **[FSC]**

Take 3g of vitamin C with bioflavonoids daily, along with bromelain which is anti-inflammatory and aids digestion. • **[S]**

Glucosamine sulphate (*for details, see* **Osteo-arthritis Supplements**. *See also* **Fats You Need to Eat**.)

Algesic cream contains an ayurvedic herb, boswellia, that is effective in reducing pain and inflammation. • **[HN]**

HINTS for all types of arthritis

Many readers have accredited relief to the following items:

Collacept I and II – a powdered supplement containing collagen from chickens, acerola cherry, vitamin C and gelatine. Many readers report relief from osteo and rheumatoid arthritis after a few weeks. For details call 0181 390 9362.

Green Barley Plus and SeaCare, which alkalize the system. For details call 0181 504 2755, or send an SAE to: Nature's Wealth, 40 Forrest Way, Woodford Wells, Essex IG8 0QS.

Sufferers of rheumatoid arthritis should consider the Immuno Test (£295). Removing all food allergens may reverse symptoms in many types of arthritis. For details call 01435 882 880.

Wearing magnets has given relief from the pain. For details of the magnetic aids, send an SAE to: Acar-Sud, Westfield House, Hampton Court Road, East Molesey, Surrey KT8 9BX.

Homeopathic remedies, acupuncture, Chinese herbs, taking stabilized aloe vera juice or consult a qualified nutritionist (*see* **Useful Information** *for further details*). The Chinese exercise regimes of Tai Chi or Qigong have helped many sufferers as they are easy to practise, even with severely impaired mobility. Rheumatoid seems to be affected by stress, so make sure you stay as calm as possible (*see* **Stress**).

For help, ideas and counselling on arthritis call: Arthritis Care on their Freephone Helpline between 12 to 4pm, Monday to Friday, 0800 289170.

For the Arthritic Association, call 0171 491 0233. This charity provides very good dietary advice – yearly membership costs £6.

Reading
Say No to Arthritis by Patrick Holford, £5.95, ION Press.
Arthritis by Stephen Terrass, £4.99, Thorsons.
Arthritis – Cause and Control by Dr Barton-Wright, £2.50, Bunter Bird Publishing. To order call 0181 874 1130.
The Natural Way With Arthritis and Rheumatism by Pat Young, £3.99, Element Books.

ASTHMA (*see also* **Allergies**)
Asthma is a disease which affects the airways leading to periods of wheezing and shortness of breath. Potential triggers for asthma include exercise, cold air, animal hair,

dust, pollution, food, stress, pollen, cigarette smoke and medication such as aspirin. Stop smoking and stay away from cigarette smoke (passive smoking) at all times.

Diet

Avoid mucus-forming foods like cow's milk and cheese, white bread, cakes, chocolate and biscuits. Eat wholemeal bread, brown rice and pasta, and try non-dairy rice or oat milk. There appears to be a particularly strong association between asthma and dairy products, especially in childhood. Reduce your intake of salt, junk foods, fizzy drinks, sugar, nuts and seafood. Avoid food and drink that has been preserved with sulphur, such as dried fruits, wines, beers and commercially produced salads. Vitally important in the control of asthma is the elimination of all food additives as these are often implicated in the triggering of attacks. The diet should be rich in dark green leaf and orange vegetables, garlic, onions, fresh salmon, mackerel, sardines and extra virgin olive oil. If you have a juicer, try carrot and radish juice daily. Also include linseeds, linseed oil and pumpkin seeds in the diet. (*see* **General Health Hints**).

Supplements

Take 2g of vitamin C with bioflavonoids (especially the bioflavonoid quercetin) daily to help open the airways, plus 200mg of magnesium. According to research published in *The Lancet*, low magnesium levels have been found in many patients suffering from asthma and chronic airway diseases. A multi-vitamin and mineral capsule. • **[LGF]**

The herb ginkgo biloba (100mg of standardized extract) plus essential fatty acids are also known to help asthma (*see* **Fats You Need To Eat**).

To help heal a leaky gut, which often contributes to asthma, take N-acetyl glucosamine (NAG), an amino sugar. • **[BC]**

Herbetom is a concentrated blend of herbal extracts and

nutrients which are known for their action on mucous membranes of the respiratory tract. The formula was developed and tested in Spanish clinics and was found to be effective in several clinical trials. • **[NC]**

Reading
New Self Help For Asthma by Leon Chaitow, £2.99, Thorsons.
The Asthma Action Plan by John Chapman, £5.99, Thorsons.
The Natural Way With Asthma by Roy Ridgeway, £3.99, Element Books.

Hints
To check for food and environmental allergens, consult a kinesiologist who can determine what foods and environmental agents you should avoid (*see* **Useful Information** *for further details*).

Potter's make a herbal mixture containing hore hound, pleurisy root, senega and lobelia called Chest Mixture, which is available from all good health stores.

Many asthmatics benefit from tuition in proper breathing techniques. Correct breathing is an integral part of yoga and is also useful for stress reduction too.

Colonic irrigation, homeopathy and consulting a nutritionist have proved helpful for many sufferers. In the case of children, homeopathy has proved especially helpful, but be sure to consult a qualified doctor who is also a homeopath (*see* **Useful Information** *for further details*).

Honeywell make a room air filter called Envirocare which removes all known airborne allergens. For details call Essential Systems on 01344 874573.

Consult the Asthma Helpline 0345 010203 9am–9pm.

National Asthma Campaign Information packs are available by calling 0171 971 0414.

ATHLETE'S FOOT

Athlete's foot is caused by a fungal infection of the skin and is characterized by itching, soreness and cracking of the skin, especially between the toes and on the soles. The condition is sometimes transmitted in public places where people walk barefoot. Fungal infections thrive in moist atmospheres, so wear socks made from natural fibres such as cotton or wool that allow your feet to breathe. The feet should be washed thoroughly and carefully dried. Persistent athlete's foot is almost always associated with an overgrowth of candida yeast in the gut and the only way to clear it up for good is to go on a strict anti-candida diet for a period of at least a month (*see* **Candida**).

Diet

Avoid any foods that contain refined sugar as this feeds yeast in the body. Try Pau D'arco tea from your health shop which has natural anti-fungal properties. Keep your diet really clean and eat lots of wholegrains, like brown rice, along with pulses, fresh fruit and plenty of raw or steamed vegetables (*see* **General Health Hints**).

Supplements

Tea tree oil is a powerful anti-fungal agent. Add a few drops to your bath water or foot bath and soak your feet for ten minutes before bed each night.

Take two acidophilus capsules daily to restore healthy bacteria in the gut which is essential in fighting fungal infections. Sprinkling between the toes with the contents of an acidophilus capsule can help provide topical relief from the discomfort of athlete's foot.

Dab the affected areas with liquid garlic and take the odourless tablets internally. • **[Q]**

Cervagyn cream, which contains acidophilus, can also be applied to the affected areas. • **[BC]**

Hints
Use Nutribiotic natural foot powder which contains Citricidal, plus tea tree oil which can be applied neat to the affected area with a cotton bud. Always wash hands afterwards. A skin spray made by Higher Nature is available from good health stores.

BACK PAIN

Back pain accounts for the loss of twenty million working days each year in Britain and affects about 80% of people at some point in their lives. In simple terms, the back can be thought of as a column made up of 33 pieces of bone called vertebrae. The back is strengthened by ligaments, which run the length of the spine, and is supported by muscles which attach to the vertebrae through tendons. Most back pain occurs in the lower part of the back called the lumbar region. Pain in this area is often due to damage to an intervertebral disc causing inflammation in, or around, the nerves that run up and down the spine, more commonly referred to as a slipped disc. Occasionally, pain in the back has nothing to do with the spine. Pain felt in the loins, for instance, is very often due to a problem in the kidneys.

Supplements
Glucosamine sulphate, an amino acid sugar, helps to restore the thick, gelatinous nature of the fluids and tissues around the joints and in-between the vertebrae. To be effective, try three x 500mg daily for three weeks. Thereafter take two daily for nine months, plus an antioxidant formula such as Solgar's Advanced Antioxidant Complex capsules. Take 3g of vitamin C daily to aid tissue healing. • [NC]

Magnesium Malate has proved useful for pain relief. Also Ligazyme (containing calcium, vitamin C, bromelain and magnesium aspartate) developed by a chiropractor to help with skeletal problems. Take one mega GLA daily, an essential fatty acid which is converted in the body to nutrients known to have anti-inflammatory properties. • [BC]

Reading
The Natural Way With Back Pain by Helena Bridge, £3.99, Element Books.
Treat Your Own Back by Robin McKenzie, £7.99. To order, call ProCare Medipost Ltd on 0161 678 0233.
Painstoppers by Donald Norfolk, £10.40, Reward Books. Available to order from 0171 436 5122.

Hints
Back pain often has its root in poor posture. This is compounded by the fact that we now tend to lead very sedentary lives, which weakens the supporting structures in the back and makes them much more prone to injury. Also much severe back pain is caused by muscle spasm. Before agreeing to any surgery, always consult a chiropractor or osteopath for a second opinion (*see* **Useful Information** *for further details*). Severe and persistent back pain should be reported to your doctor.

Acupuncture is known to help in many cases. For general back maintenance, yoga can be very beneficial as it improves flexibility and strengthens the spine and improves posture, protecting it from injury in the long term. The Alexander Technique teaches individuals how to maintain back and general health through better posture (*see* **Useful Information** *for further details*). Exercise is important too. It is generally accepted that swimming is the best form of exercise, because although the back muscles are worked, they are protected from jarring by the support given by the water.

Many readers report good results from using a wooden 'backstretcher' for ten minutes each day. For a brochure, send a large SAE to: The Ultimate Backstretcher, 63 New Inn Lane, Guildford, Surrey GU4 7HT.

Empulse is a pulsed electromagnetic treatment, the setting of which is governed by an analysis of the brain's electrical activity. It is a non-invasive, non-drug based preventative treatment. Further details are available from: MDI Ltd, 17 Owen Road, Diss, Norfolk IP22 3ER or call 01379 644234.

An excellent video which is packed with sensible, easy to understand advice is *Your Back: An Owner's Guide To Its Care and Maintenance* by Professor Diane Newham, England's first Professor of Physiotherapy, £12.44 inc p&p from Eye Eye Ltd on 0171 700 3555.

For a large information pack, send £2 to the Back Pain Association, 16 Elm Tree Road, Teddington, Middlesex TW11 8ST, or call their helpline on 0181 977 5474.

BAD BREATH (*see* Halitosis)

BEREAVEMENT

Because I have written regularly about life after death, I have received many letters from people who have lost a loved one. Their desolation and feelings of isolation are heartbreaking. I have a strong belief in life after death, which definitely has nothing to do with the occult or any particular religion. After my mother died, I derived great comfort from imagining her near me and by talking to her.

It is important for you to be able to share your feelings with someone who has gone through a similar experience. On a person's death we all wish there were things we had said and done, regrets, guilt and the seemingly endless emotion of desperately wanting to see that loved one again. It is normal to grieve for a few months, but as time passes the hurt should lessen a little. Crying lets out the emotion as tears shed in trauma contain a high level of stress chemicals, so a good cry really can bring relief. Professional counselling is invaluable if you find you cannot let go and the depression does not lift.

It is easy to forget to eat properly under such painful conditions, but remember that by making an effort to look after yourself with a balanced diet and exercise, this will help you to cope.

Supplements
Try Bach Rescue Remedy, Emergency Essence by Jan De Vries or homeopathic *ignatia*, available from all good health stores.

Take a multi-vitamin and mineral supplement at such times when motivation and appetite are reduced. The herb St John's Wort is effective in helping to ease depression, if taken regularly. • [NC]

Reading
A Time to Grieve by Carol Staudacher, £9.99, Souvenir Press. *Testimony of Light* by Helen Graves, £5.95, Neville Spearman. To order, call Watkins Books on 0171 836 2182. *Embraced by the Light* by Betty J Eadie, £4.99, Aquarian Press. *Bereavement* by Ursula Markham, £4.99, Element Books.

Hints
Cruse Bereavement Care, a charity founded in 1959, which has 180 branches in the UK. For further information, write to Cruse Bereavement Care, 126 Sheen Road, Richmond, Surrey TW9 1UR or call 0181 940 4818.

Compassionate Friends is a nation-wide organization of bereaved parents offering friendship and understanding.

Also a quarterly Newsletter, Postal Library and a range of leaflets, and offers befriending rather than counselling. For further information, contact: The Compassionate Friends, 53 North Street, Bristol BS3 1EN. Helpline 01179 539639.

BLADDER (*see* **Cystitis, Incontinence, Prostate**)

BLEEDING GUMS

Bleeding gums can be caused by excessive brushing but they are more often a sign of gum disease such as chronic infection, or a deficiency of vitamin C in the diet. If you tend to bruise easily and have bleeding gums, suspect vitamin C deficiency. Make sure you see an oral hygienist and a dentist at least twice each year for a thorough clean and check up.

Diet
The bacteria which cause chronic gum infections thrive on sugar, so this should be kept to a minimum in the diet. Eating plenty of foods which are rich in vitamin C and bioflavonoids like fruits and vegetables, will help prevent any deficiency of these nutrients (*see* **General Health Hints**).

Supplements
Two Colleginase (containing vitamin C, rutin, hesperidin, silica, vitamins A and D) all of which strengthen the tiny blood vessels in the gums. Take 30–60mg of CoEnzyme Q10 daily (not to be taken if pregnant) – very effective in treating gum disease by strengthening the gum tissues. If the gums are bleeding badly, for two weeks take extra vitamin C, up to 3g daily. • **[BC]**

Hints
Practise good daily dental hygiene by using a floss and a natural tea tree mouthwash. Clean your teeth and gums daily using a water jet and appliance, adding a few drops of tea tree oil and one drop of clove oil, which is an excellent antiseptic, to the warm water. Water Tooth Cleaners are available from large chemists. Use a good herbal toothpaste like Sarakan, Blackmores or Nutribiotic.

BLEPHARITIS (*see* Eye Problems)

BODY HAIR, EXCESSIVE (Hirsutism)
In women, excess hair due to hormonal imbalance is usually due to an excess of male hormones called androgens. These can be produced by the ovaries or the adrenal glands. You should consult your doctor if you have unexplained excess body hair.

Diet
Eat more hormone-regulating foods like soya bean curd (tofu) and organic vegetables like cauliflower, broccoli and artichokes (*see* General Health Hints).

Supplements
The herbs, dong quai or agnus castus, when taken for a few months help to regulate hormones and are usually effective for resolving excess body hair. • [BLK]
Black cohosh has been used during and after menopause to inhibit and reverse facial hair growth in women. • [FSC]

Hints

Women who grow excessive body hair may be short of progesterone, which helps balance the male hormones that women also make in small quantities. Many women don't ovulate regularly (but still have periods) due to stress, excess pollution in the environment and foods containing herbicides which have an oestrogen affect on the body. As progesterone is only produced after ovulation or during pregnancy, progesterone deficiency is becoming more common and hairy legs and chins are one sign. Natural progesterone, made from yams in a cream called Pro-Gest, can reduce hairiness when used for some time. It is available by prescription in the UK (but freely available in America). For further information on this send £2 to: The Natural Progesterone Information Service, BCM 4315, London WC1N 3XX.

Reading
Balancing Hormones Naturally by Kate Neil. £4.95, ION Press. To order, call 0181 877 9993.

BODY ODOUR

Body odour is usually due to bacteria on the skin, which turn substances in sweat into foul-smelling chemicals. Sometimes, just as with bad breath, body odour can be the sign of internal toxicity. It can rarely be caused by eating spicy or strong-flavoured foods such as garlic which are eliminated to some degree through the skin.

Diet
Personal hygiene is of obvious importance in combating body odour, but eating a clean diet rich in fruits, vegetables and wholegrain cereals will also help. It is important not to

become constipated, as this can add to toxicity in the body. Drink between six or eight glasses of bottled or filtered water each day. Dairy products and meat are the foods most likely to putrefy in the gut and cause toxicity, and these should be avoided.

Supplements
Incomplete digestion of foods can lead to foods putrefying in the gut so anything that improves digestion can help if this is a factor (*see* **Acid Stomach** *for tips on digestion*). Taking a digestive enzyme capsule with meals can also be beneficial, along with two acidophilus capsules each day, which help maintain healthy bacteria in the gut.

Deficiency of zinc is sometimes related to excessive perspiration, so take a high potency multi-vitamin and mineral to support the whole system daily. • **[LGF]**

Green food supplements, such as blue-green algae, spirulina and chlorella, contain high levels of chlorophyll which counteracts odour and bacteria.

Reading
Food Combining in 30 Days by Kathryn Marsden, £4.99, Thorsons.
New Self-help Body Odour, Leon Chaitow, £7.99, Thorsons.

Hints
If persistent, body odour may indicate liver dysfunction, digestive problems and/or yeast infections, which are probably best investigated by a qualified nutritionist or a doctor who is also a nutritionist (*see* **Useful Information** *for details*).

Try PitRok – a natural odourless mineral salt deodorant which prevents bacterial growth without the use of harsh chemicals or aluminium. Just wet the crystal and glide it over the skin. Available from most health food shops or call PitRok on 0181 563 1120.

BOILS

A boil is caused by an acute bacterial infection of a hair follicle. Boils are often painful and tender, and may be accompanied by a slight fever. Recurrent boils are often associated with a poor diet, poor immune function and are more common in diabetics.

Diet

The diet should be kept clean, with an emphasis on fresh fruits, vegetables and whole grains. Food which tend to suppress the immune system like sugar and refined carbohydrates such as white bread, biscuits and shop-bought cakes should be kept to an absolute minimum (*see* **General Health Hints**).

Supplements

Zinc can be an effective treatment for recurrent boils by stimulating the immune system and skin healing. Take 45mg daily for one month. Take 3g of vitamin C, plus a natural beta-carotene complex and 5,000iu of vitamin A daily for six weeks. Garlic is antiseptic and cleansing, along with a B complex. • **[NC]**

Reading

Super Skin by Kathryn Marsden, £5.99, Thorsons.

Hints

Tea Tree Oil, a natural antiseptic, is excellent for boils and can be applied neat, if required.

Make sure you get plenty of exercise, which helps detoxify the skin, and wash as soon as possible after exercise. Saunas help to clear blocked pores and drain toxins from the body.

✳ ❈ ✳

BREAST PAIN AND TENDERNESS (*see also* **Cancer of the Breast**)

Breast pain and tenderness is a common symptom of pre-menstrual syndrome (PMS) when the breasts can become increasingly swollen and tender prior to menstruation. Breast pain is often associated with other symptoms such as fluid retention, abdominal bloating and an excess of the hormone oestrogen. Wearing a bra for more than 12 hours a day can prevent toxins draining from lymph nodes in this area. Breast tenderness in the first three months of pregnancy is quite common. If breast tenderness is present for most of the month, or if it is severe, then consult your doctor. **If you find any lumps in your breasts, see your GP immediately.**

Diet

Avoid salt in the diet which can exacerbate fluid retention known to exacerbate breast tenderness. Alcohol and caffeine (particularly coffee) should be minimized as these can increase breast pain. Coffee can be replaced with barley coffee, dandelion coffee, herb and fruit teas. If you want to drink decaffeinated coffee, choose one which states it has been decaffeinated using the Swiss water method, as other processes use potentially harmful chemicals.

Soya products like tofu and vegetables such as cabbage, broccoli and cauliflower contain plant oestrogens known to have a balancing and beneficial effect on hormones. Kombu seaweed or kelp both contain iodine known to relieve mastitis-type breast pain.

Supplements

Take 400mg of magnesium daily, (a muscle relaxant). Also 300iu of vitamin E, as studies have shown this supplement to be useful in reducing breast pain and tenderness. Take 1g of evening primrose oil, taken, three times daily, as essential fatty acids help reduce breast tenderness associated with PMS and a multi-vitamin for women like Femforte. • **[BC]**

Red clover tea is an excellent blood cleanser, as are Blue Flag Root tablets by Gerard House. Available from all good health shops.

Reading
Your Breasts: What Every Woman Needs To Know by Brian Butler, £9.95, TASK Books, PO Box 359A, Surbiton, Surrey KT5 8YP or call 0181 399 3215.

Hints
If, after three months, there is no improvement on the above regime, see a qualified nutritionist who is also a doctor (*see* **Useful Information** *for details*).

Sometimes breast pain is due to an imbalance between oestrogen and progesterone which causes tender breasts and breast cysts, and is often called fibrocystic breast disease. It is becoming increasingly common because of the high levels of oestrogen pollutants we are exposed to. Using a natural progesterone cream, such as Pro-Gest cream, may reduce the cysts and tenderness in a few months. You need a prescription for Pro-Gest in the UK (but not abroad). For further information, send £2 to: The Natural Progesterone Information Service, BCM 4315, London WC1N 3XX. As with any hormonal treatment there are potential hazards with progesterone and it is wise only to use it if you have been shown to really need it. Diagnostech is a specialised laboratory service which offers hormone measurements based on saliva samples. For details, send an SAE to The Cottage, Lakeside Centre, 180 Lifford Lane, Kings Norton, Birmingham, B30 3NT.

Lymphatic drainage massage is known to improve drainage, thereby reducing swelling and pain (*see* **MLD [Manual Lymphatic Drainage]** *in* **Useful Information**).

Regular exercise improves circulation and aids drainage of the lymph system. Rebounders (mini-trampolines) are wonderful for this problem, as is any vigorous exercise such as fast walking, swimming or dancing.

BRUISING

Bruising is caused by blood leaking from damaged blood vessels into the tissues of the skin. Bruising is a normal process, but in some individuals the slightest trauma can lead to painful and unsightly bruising. Excessive bruising is often due to a deficiency of vitamin C and bioflavonoids in the diet.

Diet
The diet should be rich in foods which are high in vitamin C and bioflavonoids including fresh fruits, particularly citrus fruits and vegetables (*see* **General Health Hints**).

Supplements
Take 2g of vitamin C complex, which includes bioflavonoids to help strengthen capillaries. Bromelain is an anti-inflammatory flavonoid derived from pineapple, so if you have bad bruising take 500mg three times daily on an empty stomach plus a high potency multi-vitamin. • **[FSC]**

Reading
Arnica The Wonder Herb by Phyllis Speight, £3.75. Available from Nelsons Mail Order, 73 Duke Street, London W1 or call 0171 495 2404.

Hints
Arnica is a homeopathic remedy which, as a cream, helps with healing in the locality of the bruise. Taken orally,

arnica can also be effective in reducing the impact of general trauma, including surgery. When I recently had surgery which had previously caused a huge amount of swelling, I took arnica tablets under my tongue twice before the operation and every two hours for two days post operatively and had virtually no swelling!

BURNS, Minor
First degree burns affect the very top layer of the skin; second degree burns leave blisters but usually heal without scarring. Third degree burns affect the full thickness of the skin, leaving it looking charred or white. These burns need urgent medical attention to reduce risk of infection and minimize scarring. If you are in any doubt at all, see your doctor.

Diet
Eat good quality protein like organic chicken, fresh fish, pulses and beans, as protein is essential for tissue healing in the initial stages (*see* **General Health Hints**).

Supplements
The herb gotu kola has been historically used for wound healing and burns. It works as a result of its effect on cells and tissues participating in the process of healing, particularly in connective tissue. Gotu kola can be used both internally and topically. Also take 2g of vitamin C with bioflavonoids daily plus 300iu of natural vitamin E. A beta carotene complex plus B complex and 30–60mg of zinc, all good for skin healing and to boost the immune system. • **[FSC]**

Hints

Studies in Bombay have shown that when fresh potato peelings are placed on burns, the wounds heal more quickly and infection is reduced. Run cold water initially over the burn. You can bathe the burn in cold water for up to 30 minutes, if necessary. Dry with a clean sterile dressing. Aloe vera gel or calendula cream can be applied topically. Nutraderm, a vitamin C and A cream, can be applied topically to aid healing of minor burns. For details call 01435 882880. Once healing is underway, pierce a vitamin E capsule and apply directly to the affected area to promote healing.

BURSITIS

Bursitis is inflammation of the bursa, the sac-like membrane containing the fluid responsible for lubricating all joints in the body. Most commonly it affects the shoulder, elbow, hip and knee, and causes severe pain, particularly on movement.

Diet

Avoid caffeine and alcohol, which increase inflammation in the body. Also, cut down on foods which tend to lead to excess acidity in the body such as bread, dairy produce and meat. Eat more foods which are alkalizing, such as fruits (but not plums, rhubarb or oranges), vegetables and millet. It helps to include fresh ginger in the diet as this has natural anti-inflammatory properties. Ginger tea can be easily made by steeping slices of root ginger in hot water, a good way to enjoy the benefits of ginger. (*See* **General Health Hints**).

Supplements

2g of vitamin C with bioflavonoids helps to heal and reduce inflammation. Boswellic Acid Complex (a herbal supplement containing boswellic acid, turmeric, bilberry extract and ginger) which has anti-inflammatory properties. For optimum anti-inflammatory effect, take this complex with Mega EPA 1,000, a fish oil concentrate and OptiZinc. Ligazyme (containing calcium, vitamin C, bromelain and magnesium aspartate), a dietary supplement designed by an osteopath to provide optimal nutrition for the musculo-skeletal system. • [BC]

Glucosamine sulphate, an amino acid sugar which helps to restore the thick gelatinous fluids and tissues around the joints and vertebrae. To be effective, try three 500mg capsules daily for three weeks, thereafter two daily for three months. • [NC]

Reading
Arthritis by Michael Murray ND, £9.95, Prima Press. Available from 0171 436 5122.
Arthritis by Stephen Terrass, £4.99, Thorsons.

Hints
Apply a bag of frozen peas wrapped in a tea towel to ice the painful area for ten minutes every few hours. This really does help to reduce inflammation and pain. Compress the area with an elastic bandage to limit swelling. Elevate the affected area above the level of the heart to encourage drainage of fluids out of the injured area.

Many acupuncturists believe that bursitis results from muscle spasms which pull joints out of line. Treatment consists of releasing muscle spasm by inserting fine acupuncture needles into the muscle trigger points. Gentle aromatherapy massage using oils like marjoram and geranium can also help to relieve the pain (*see* **Useful Information** *for further details*).

CANCER (*see also* Cancer of The Breast)

At the heart of the cancer causing process are destructive substances called free radicals. These harmful substances can damage cells and suppress the immune system. Substances called 'antioxidants' (such as vitamins A, C and E, beta carotene and the minerals zinc and selenium), have been shown in many scientific studies to neutralize free radicals and inhibit the growth of cancer cells. Essentially, the more antioxidant nutrients there are in the body, the less chance there is of getting cancer. Chemicals in the environment have also been implicated in the development of cancer. Many chemicals, such as herbicides and pesticides, mimic the effects of oestrogen in the body and certain tumours, such as cancers of the breast and prostate, seem to be triggered or accelerated by oestrogen.

The Alternative Anti-Cancer Prevention Diet

Avoid fried food. This is a good way to cut down on your exposure to free radicals. Boil, steam or bake, eating most of your food raw or lightly cooked. Try 'steam-frying' food using a watered-down soya sauce, plus herbs or spices for taste. Barbecued and char-grilled foods, especially if rather fatty, are also best avoided because they contain relatively high concentrations of a range of cancer-causing substances called carcinogens.

Minimize pollution. Anything that is combusted produces free radicals. So the less time you spend exposed to car exhaust and other people's smoke, the better.

Eat broccoli, carrots and soya. These three foods have been found to contain anti-cancer chemicals. Soya and broccoli contain substances that counteract hormone excesses associated with breast cancer. Carrots are rich in beta-carotene, high levels of which mean a low risk of cancer. Put two carrots, two heads of broccoli, half a pack of tofu (soya bean curd), a teaspoon of vegetable stock and some water in the blender for a delicious immune-boosting soup. Add soya milk if you want it creamy and spices if you like it hot. Heat and serve.

Eat organically as much as possible. Carrots, lettuce and many other healthy foods are overloaded with pesticides that are associated with an increased risk of cancer. So, whenever possible, eat organic. Throw away the outer leaves when preparing non-organic vegetables like cabbage or lettuce. Just one serving of cabbage each week can help reduce the risk of colon cancer.

Eat at least three pieces of fruit a day. Vitamin C and natural beta-carotene are potent anti-cancer nutrients. These anti-oxidants protect your body cells from the damage that initiates the development of cancer. Fresh fruit contains lots of vitamin C. Red and orange coloured fruits, such as oranges, apricots or watermelon are loaded with beta-carotene. Eat fresh fruit as a snack throughout the day.

Eat wholefoods, nuts, beans and seeds. Anything in its whole form, such as oats, brown rice, lentils, almonds or sunflower seeds are high in the essential anti-cancer minerals zinc and selenium. These protect the body from free radicals.

Supplement your diet with anti-oxidant nutrients. Many scientific studies have found low rates of cancer in people who have high levels of anti-oxidants in their blood. The anti-oxidant nutrients are primarily vitamin A, a carotenoid complex that includes lycopene derived from natural sources, vitamin C, vitamin E and the minerals zinc and selenium.

Minimize alcohol. Alcohol is associated with an increased risk of cancer. Red wine does, however, contain anti-oxidant nutrients called polyphenols which are associated with a reduced risk of heart disease. One glass a day is the recommended maximum. Red grape juice contains the same anti-oxidants without the alcohol.

Healthy oils

Organic flax seed oil helps to boost the immune and digestive systems. Omega Nutrition's Flax Seed is available from good health stores and must be kept in the fridge. Take one tablespoon daily in any freshly made vegetable juice (*for further details, see* **Fats You Need To Eat**).

Reading

Cancer The Positive Approach by Karol Sikora and Hilary Thomas, £8.99, Thorsons.
Cancer and Its Nutritional Therapies by Dr Richard Passwater, £12.50. To order, call 0181 877 9993.
Alternatives in Cancer Therapy by Pelton and Overholster, £11.40, Simon and Schuster. To order, call 0171 436 5122.
Cancer: Another Opinion by Dr John Stirling, £9.95, BioMed Publications. To order, call BioMed on 0121 433 4569. The most up-to-date book covering all conventional and alternative methods relating to the treatment of cancer. Well worth a read.
Nutrition and Cancer: State of the Art by Sandra Goodman PhD, £7.99. To order, call 0117 983 8851.

Hints for cancer patients receiving treatment

If you are already undergoing any type of cancer therapy, Dr Rosy Daniel (the Medical Director of the Bristol Cancer Help Centre) says that nutrition is vital to help bring back up the white blood cell count. She advises patients to eat plenty of organic fresh fruit and vegetables along with wholefoods like brown rice and brown bread. All animal fats should be avoided. A daily bottle of Guinness helps to improve blood count as it contains iron and folic acid. She also recommends that cancer patients take a good anti-oxidant formula which contains vitamin C, natural beta-carotene complex, zinc and selenium. Dr Daniel stresses that fear drains energy levels and advocates any therapy that can reduce anxiety, such as spiritual healing, relaxation exercises, visualization, acupuncture or homeopathy.

Maitake Mushrooms available in capsule form have been shown to stimulate the immune system and seem to reduce the effects of chemotherapy. For details ask at your local health store or call 0171 436 5122.

There are many associations which offer help, counselling and advice including Bristol Cancer Help Centre, Grove House, Cornwallis Grove, Clifton, Bristol BS8 4PG. Patient Helpline 01179 743216.

CANCER OF THE BREAST – Prevention of

One woman in twelve in the UK develops breast cancer. Orthodox HRT, the Pill and too much saturated fat seems to increase the risk of breast cancer. Breast cancer is more common in the overweight and obese. Many scientists now believe that chemicals in the environment such as herbicides and pesticides can promote the development of breast cancer by mimicking the effects of oestrogen in the body.

Recent studies in the USA have found that women who wear tightly-fitting bras for more than 14 hours a day are 50% more likely to develop breast cancer. Tightly fitting bras obstruct the lymph drainage system in the breasts, which is important for the removal of toxins from breast tissue and the efficient functioning of the immune system.

Diet
Nature provides natural anti-cancer agents in certain foods, predominantly organic fruit, vegetables and seeds. These are rich in beta-carotene (levels of natural carotenes are often low in cancer patients), vitamin C and E and minerals like zinc and selenium. Red/orange foods like carrots or tomatoes are rich in beta-carotene, which is converted naturally into vitamin A in the body. Mauve/blue foods, like berries and beetroot are also rich in anti-oxidants. Eat

plenty of organic apples which are rich in pectin and fibre. Lack of fibre is linked to cancer, so eat more oat-based cereals, raw linseeds and brown rice.

Reduce meat and cows' milk which often contain anti-biotic residues. Also non-organic vegetables and fruits are often covered in pesticide residues. Broccoli and soya products such as tofu contain specific compounds that help to correct hormonal imbalances and can also help protect against breast cancer.

Supplements
An anti-oxidant complex that contains mixed carotenoids, vitamins A, C and E, selenium, zinc, copper, manganese.

30–60mg CoEnzyme Q10 which boosts the immune system. Imbalances in fatty acids are linked to an increase in breast cancer, therefore take an essential fatty acid complex containing Omega 3 and 6 oils (*see* **Fats You Need to Eat**).

Reading
Your Breasts: What Every Woman Needs To Know, by Brian Butler, £9.95, TASK Books, PO Box 359A, Surbiton, Surrey KT5 8YP. Tel: 0181 399 3215.

Breast Cancer, What You Should Know and May Not Be Told About Prevention, Diagnosis and Treatment by Dr Steven Austin and Cathy Hitchcock, £8.99, Prima Press. To order, call Bookpoint on 01235 400400.

Cancer and Its Nutritional Therapies by Dr Richard Passwater, £12.50. To order, call 0181 877 9993.

Hints
High stress levels are associated with breast cancer – make sure you get plenty of exercise which reduces the tendency towards stress.

Bristol Cancer Help Centre, Grove House, Cornwallis Grove, Clifton, Bristol BS8 4PG. Patient Helpline 01179 743216 between 9am–5pm Monday–Friday.

✳ ❋ ✳

CANDIDA

Candida albicans is a yeast that is responsible for the condition known as thrush. It is a common misconception that candida can only live in the vagina. In fact, the main reservoir for candida is in the gut. Normally, relatively low levels of candida are present in the gut as they are balanced by large amounts of healthy bacteria which help keep the yeast in check. Problems occur when yeast starts to overgrow in the gut which can ultimately lead to a variety of symptoms such as bloating, wind and constipation and/or diarrhoea. Candida can make the lining of the gut leaky which increases the risk of food sensitivity (*see* **Allergies**). Candida affects men and women alike but is more common in women.

Outside the gut, candida is associated with symptoms such as itching, fatigue, food cravings, headaches, and general aches and pains. Another misconception is that you can't have candida if you don't have thrush. In fact, the majority of women with a candida problem do not have thrush.

Diet

The secret to reducing candida is by starving it out of the gut. Yeast loves sugar and refined carbohydrates such as white bread, white rice and pasta. These foods should be eliminated from the diet for at least two months. Fruit, because it is fermentable, if not eliminated temporarily, should be cut to a couple of pieces per day. It is also necessary to avoid foods containing yeast. These include bread, cheese, alcohol, yeast extract spreads, stock cubes and gravy mixes, dried fruit, mushrooms, soy sauce and vinegar. The diet should be based around fresh vegetables, wholegrains like brown rice and whole-wheat pasta, meat and fish. Live, low-fat natural yoghurt contains bacterial cultures which may help restore beneficial bacteria in the gut in the short term.

Supplements

Take two bio-acidophilus capsules daily to replace the good bacteria in the gut, plus garlic to help eliminate the candida. Mycopryl, made from time-released caprylic acid, to inhibit yeast overgrowth. **(Do not take if pregnant or suffering intestinal ulcers.)** For more resistant cases, take two Candicidin daily (**not if pregnant**), a powerful anti-fungal agent which helps rid the entire system of candida. • **[BC]**

The herb Pau D'arco has anti-fungal properties and can be taken daily either in capsule form or as a tea while the condition lasts. • **[S]**

Reading

Could Yeast Be Your Problem? by Leon Chaitow, £3.99. To order, call 0181 877 9993.

Candida and Thrush, a booklet by Dr George Lewith, £2.95 plus p&p from BioMed Publications Ltd, 16 Court Oak Grove, Harborne, Birmingham B32 2HR.

The Practical Guide To Candida by Jane McWhirter explains the condition clearly and includes a directory of practitioners in the UK who treat candida naturopathically – £8.75, and available from the Green Library, 9 Rickett Street, Fulham, London SW6 1RU.

Hints

For further help and advice on candida infections, send an SAE and £2 to: The Candida Support Group, 10 Burghley Road, London NW5 1UE.

Recent research indicates that people who have persistent and chronic candida may have intestinal parasites known as flukes. Doctor Hulda Clark from Canada has shown that a herbal combination containing wormwood, tincture of black walnut hull and cloves, plus the amino acids ornithine and arginine helps eliminate parasites successfully. For details of this candida cleanse formula call G&G Food Supplies on 01342 312811.

CARPAL TUNNEL SYNDROME (CTS)

This syndrome is characterized by pain, numbness or tingling in the thumb, index and middle finger and the thumb side of the ring finger. The condition is caused by compression of a nerve that runs under a band of tissue in the wrist. CTS is more common in women and can be associated with an underactive thyroid, pregnancy, weight gain and arthritis.

Diet
Because this condition is associated with fluid retention, it is wise to avoid salt in food preparation or at the table. Avoid all shop-bought cakes and pre-packaged foods which are often high in salt, fat and sugar (*see* **General Health Hints**).

Supplements
A regular intake of vitamin B6 and B complex is known to help this condition if taken daily for at least three months. Ginkgo Plus (bilberry concentrate and vitamin C as potassium ascorbate) supports the health of the circulatory system. Ligazyme (containing B6 and bromelain) is a natural anti-inflammatory supplement to help support the ligaments. Colleginase (containing vitamin C, rutin, hesperidin, cellulase, silica, vitamins A and D) helps strengthen connective tissue plus Mega EPA 1,000, a concentrated fish oil to help reduce inflammation. • [BC]

Reading
Carpal Tunnel Syndrome and Overuse Injuries by Tammy Crouch & Michael Madden, £13.25, North Atlantic Books. Available from 0171 436 5122.

Hints
If symptoms are severe, buy a wrist splint which is available

from good pharmacies. Sleeping heavily on your side, with your wrists tucked under you, can also cause this condition. If you wake up with numb hands, immediately shake them and give them a quick massage to restore circulation.

CATARACTS

A cataract is a clouding of the normally clear and transparent lens of the eye. When a cataract develops, the lens becomes cloudy like a frosted window and is accompanied by gradual loss of vision. Ultraviolet light (too much sun), a poor diet, some chronic diseases such as diabetes and the use of certain drugs including steroids can all cause cataracts.

Diet
The most important protecting nutrients are vitamins C and E and the mineral selenium. These are found in fruits, vegetables and seeds like sunflower, pumpkin and linseeds (*see also* **General Health Hints**).

Supplements
Bilberry Ginkgo Eyebright Complex. Bilberry is rich in flavonoids which improve overall eye function and along with ginkgo benefits circulation and protects eyes from free radical damage (this complex also includes carotenoids, vitamins A, C, E and selenium). • **[S]**

Reading
The New SuperNutrition by Dr Richard Passwater, £5.99, Pocket Books. Available from 0171 436 5122.

Hints
Anyone concerned about developing cataracts should protect their eyes from bright sunlight with a pair of

sunglasses which have been verified for UV filtering ability. If you work outside, wear a sun hat to protect your eyes. UV filtering contact lenses are also available. Ask your optician for details.

CATARRH

Chronic catarrh can be caused by an allergy to an airborne allergen such as dust or the house dust mite. But more often the root cause of chronic catarrh is a sensitivity to foods like cow's milk, cheese and wheat.

Diet

As an alternative to cows' milk, cheese and yoghurt, try rice or oat milk, goats' or sheeps' milk and yoghurt. Avoid chocolate, white bread, shop bought cakes and biscuits, too much sugar and saturated fat. Keep your diet as clean as possible, eat a little of everything but keep a note of when the problem is most severe. Drink plenty of filtered water to help eliminate toxins from the body (*see* **General Health Hints**).

Supplements

Muccolyte, a complex containing vitamins A, C and D, potassium and digestive enzyme to support and maintain mucus membranes. 1g of vitamin C with bioflavonoids. • **[BC]**

Garlic is extremely cleansing for the sinuses but it must be taken regularly for at least six weeks.

The herb fenugreek is a useful expectorant made in capsule form by Solgar. Also try New Era Tissue Salts for catarrh.

Reading

Food Combining in 30 Days by Kathryn Marsden, £4.99, Thorsons.

Hints

Invest in a humidifier/air filter that is available from health stores to help keep the air in the immediate environment free of potential allergens.

Try an allergy testing like the Elisa Test from Larkhall Green Farm. Tel: 0181 874 1130 for details.

Inhale a mixture of cooled boiled water, mixed with a small amount of olive oil and a pinch of salt to wash out the sinuses. I do this by simply splashing the mixture into the palm of my hand and inhaling it. Not pleasant – but very effective!

Many people have found that lime flower tea is useful for reducing catarrh.

If your ears are blocked due to mucus, use warm ear candles which gently remove excess wax and congestion. For details, call 0171 976 6615.

The Hi-Tech Face Bath is a facial dip which clears the nose and sinuses and helps reduce infection. Aloe juice taken regularly reduces allergic reactions and improves digestion. • **[HN]**

CELLULITE

An unsightly dimpling of the skin, most commonly found on the hips and thighs. Cellulite is due to water retention plus a build up of toxins such as food additives and chemicals like pesticides which sit in our fatty tissues. As many more women than men seem to develop cellulite, there is possibly a hormonal link.

Diet

Avoid adding any salt to food or eating too much pre-packaged or tinned food which is often full of salt and additives. Use soya or rice milk instead of full fat cow's milk. Reduce saturated fat intake and use a healthy spread like Vitaquell instead of butter. Drink plenty of water and fresh organic vegetable juices to aid elimination of toxins. Eat foods rich in essential fats like linseeds, sunflower and pumpkin seeds. Use organic olive and walnut oil for salad dressings. Raw foods are particularly important, especially apples. The fibre in apples (called pectin) is excellent to help absorb and eliminate toxins (*see* **General Health Hints**).

Supplements
Dandelion complex, taken together with Echinacea Complex, helps your body to eliminate the waste tissue and stored chemicals that can contribute to cellulite by draining the liver and lymph glands. • **[BLK]**

Reading
Cellulite Revolution by Leslie Kenton, £5.99, Ebury Press.

Hints
Regular skin brushing or massage helps to 'rev' up the circulation which, in turn, will aid drainage of toxins. Plenty of exercise to encourage circulation and elimination of toxins. A three-day vegetable juice fast is useful, but check with your doctor or nutritionist before starting a fast.

CHILBLAINS
Chilblains are caused by poor circulation and are characterized by red, inflamed areas that affect the extremities, usually the toes. Chilblains usually occur when the weather is cold, because the small blood vessels in the skin naturally constrict at this time. They often become itchy or painful when the affected areas warm up. The basis of treating chilblains naturally is to improve the circulation.

Diet
Eat a diet low in saturated fat , but include a little organic olive oil and oily fish like salmon and mackerel. Avoid coffee, sugar, vinegar and red meat. Eat plenty of dark green and orange vegetables (*see* **Circulation** *and* **General Health Hints**).

Supplements
Ginkgo Plus containing potassium ascorbate, a form of vitamin C and bilberry to improve micro circulation. Citrase, made from magnesium and calcium, which aids circulation. Take three daily until the chilblains disappear. • **[BC]**

Organic Flax Seed Oil, rich in omega 3 fatty acids, is effective in reducing stickiness in blood. Take one tablespoon daily stirred into fresh vegetable or fruit juice. Cat's claw tea is excellent for capillaries and also thins the blood. B complex including niacin (B3) helps improve circulation. • **[HN]**

Hints
I suffer chilblains nearly all winter long, after having varicose veins removed years ago. The surgeon told me that I would still have plenty of veins left, but the legacy has been poor circulation. Obviously the key would have been for me to have avoided varicose veins in my youth! Keep this in mind and wear bed socks during winter months. Never wear tight-fitting shoes as this really aggravates chilblains by restricting circulation to the toes. Invest in fur-lined boots during cold weather.

Massage your feet with diluted essential oil of black pepper or rosemary to improve circulation and increase blood supply. Regular reflexology improves circulation.

Magnet Therapy – use Magnet Insoles known to improve circulation. For details, call Nikken Europa, Unit 7, Landmere Lane, Edwalton, Nottingham NG12 4DE. Tel: 01159 456595.

Sixtan Anti Cold Foot Balm based on alpine herbs and

herbal extracts to increase circulation. Available by mail order from JICA Beauty Products Ltd, 20 Island Farm Avenue, Molesey Trading Estate, West Molesey, Surrey KT8 2UZ or call 0181 979 7261. Keep on the move and get plenty of exercise like walking, swimming or skipping, especially in cold weather.

CHOLESTEROL, High and Low

Cholesterol is a type of fat which is present in our diet but is also manufactured by our body in the liver. Although too much cholesterol is a bad thing, some is essential to make cell walls, hormones and bile. Low levels of cholesterol are associated with an increased risk of depression and many women, who believe that very low fat diets are healthy, often become depressed (*see* **Fats You Need To Eat**). There are two basic types of cholesterol in the blood; high density lipoproteins (HDLs, the good cholesterol) and low density lipoproteins (LDLs, the bad cholesterol). The higher the level of cholesterol in your blood, the greater the risk of conditions such as heart disease and stroke. It is generally accepted that a cholesterol level below 5.2 mmol/l is healthy. If your level of cholesterol is higher than this, the risk of heart disease is likely to be increased. If your cholesterol level is above 6.5 mmol/l the risk of heart disease is much higher still.

Diet

Fibre can stop some of the fat being absorbed from your diet. Wheat fibre often irritates the gut, so use oat-based bran and cereals which help to reduce cholesterol levels. Eat plenty of fresh fruit and vegetables which are also rich in healthy fibre. Cut down on your consumption of saturated fat because this is the major source of cholesterol in the diet. This means eating as little red meat and dairy produce as possible. Go for low-fat versions of dairy products such as cottage cheese, skimmed or semi-skimmed milk and low-fat natural yoghurt. Try non-dairy rice or oat milk which is low in fat. Also avoid fried, processed and many pre-packaged foods like sausages and meat pies which are generally high in fat. If you eat poultry, remove the skin. Avoid butter and margarine. Non-hydrogenated spreads like SuperSpread and Vitaquell, available from good health food stores, are healthy alternatives. Use more mono-unsaturated extra virgin olive oil in the diet. Include some oily fish such as trout, salmon, mackerel, tuna or sardines in your diet as these contain fats which are protective for heart disease. Eat more tofu (soya bean curd) which is known to lower bad cholesterol.

Supplements

To help regulate your cholesterol levels, take CH192 which contains chromium polynicotinate, enzymes and niacin (vitamin B3), which all help to regulate cholesterol and reduce sugar cravings. Often sugary items are also packed with saturated fats, eg, cakes and biscuits). Also take a multi-vitamin plus a B complex daily. • [BC]

Take an acidophilus capsule daily (containing healthy bacteria) which binds fat and cholesterol in the intestines – available from good health stores – or eat low-fat, live yoghurt every day which contains acidophilus bacteria. In order for garlic to be effective on cholesterol levels, it needs to be taken regularly for twelve to eighteen months. Take 600–900mg daily in the middle of your main meal. (If you are on blood-thinning drugs, ask your GP before taking large amounts of garlic.) Lecithin granules help to emulsify fats. Take one tablespoon daily on your oat-based breakfast cereal. Lecithin is also good for memory function and controlling kidney and gall stones.

Essential fatty acids are vital for lowering bad cholesterol (*for details, see* **Fats You Need To Eat**).

Cat's claw tea is helpful for lowering cholesterol, blood pressure and helping prevent atherosclerosis. Linus Pauling, the Nobel Prize winning scientist, discovered that vitamin C and the amino acid lysine work together to reduce athero-sclerosis, lower blood pressure and lower cholesterol. • **[HN]**

Reading
Super Nutrition For a Healthy Heart by Patrick Holford, £2.50, ION Press.
The Fats We Need To Eat by Dr Jeannette Ewin, £6.99, Thorsons.
The Fats That Heal and Fats That Kill, Udo Erasmus, £14.50, Alive Books. To order call 0181 877 9993.

Hints
Regular exercise is absolutely vital for lowering cholesterol and keeping the heart healthy. With your doctor's permission, start walking for 30 minutes, increasing to one hour daily. Swimming, yoga and skipping are all excellent ways to stay fit.

CHRONIC FATIGUE (*see* **Exhaustion** *and* **ME**)

CIRCULATION (*see also* **Chilblains and Raynaud's**)
Bad circulation is one of the most common problems I deal with. Over 25% of my mail is from people suffering with circulatory problems. Common symptoms of poor circulation are cold hands, feet and leg ulcers. It's not just the extremities that may suffer; poor circulation to the brain can lead to memory loss and has been associated with

conditions such as senile dementia. Bad circulation is generally due to arteries which are either constricted or blocked with a cholesterol-like substance. Conditions like Raynaud's and chilblains are due to arterial constriction, while conditions like angina and dementia are usually due to hardening of the arteries.

Diet
Eat a good diet, low in saturated animal fats and salt. Eat oily fish at least twice a week and include linseeds, sunflower and pumpkin seeds in your diet. Drink at least six glasses of filtered water every day (*see* **General Health Hints**).

Supplements
Ginkgo Plus, a bioflavonoid complex containing gingko biloba and bilberry extract to improve micro circulation. Bio-magnesium taken regularly helps circulation as it reduces spasm in the artery walls. 200iu of vitamin E daily to reduce stickiness in the blood. 2g of vitamin C with bioflavonoids to strengthen capillaries. • **[BC]**

Organic Flax Seed Oil helps to thin the blood and strengthen capillaries. Take one tablespoon daily stirred into fresh vegetable or fruit juice. Cat's claw tea made with ginger, cardamom and cinnamon taken regularly helps to lower blood pressure. • **[HN]**

Garlic is helpful for thinning the blood. Take one tablet daily or include plenty of fresh garlic in your diet. (NB: if you are on blood-thinning drugs, have regular check-ups with your GP as you may be able to lower your drug intake once on this regime).

Hints
Add half a teaspoon of powdered mustard to a bowl of warm water and soak your feet, which will stimulate circulation.

Exercise is great for stimulating the circulation. Take a

brisk walk every day for at least 30 minutes. Any exercise that gently pounds the feet will help improve circulation; like dancing, skipping and rebounding. Stop smoking.

Reflexology and massage are excellent for people who, for health reasons, cannot manage much exercise (*see* **Useful Information** *for further details*). Alternatively, you could try an energy roller which works on the same principle as reflexology – roll bare feet for two minutes daily on the roller; this hurts initially but it gets easier! For further details, send an SAE to: Shakti Chakra, PO Box 3984, London SE12 0EJ.

COELIAC DISEASE

Sufferers of coeliac disease are sensitive to a dietary protein called gluten, which is present in wheat, oats, rye and barley. The condition causes changes in the intestinal lining which makes it very difficult for nutrients to be absorbed from the diet. Because fat is poorly absorbed, the stools tend to be pale, frothy and foul-smelling. Sufferers are also likely to be deficient in a number of nutrients. This condition often goes undiagnosed for many years.

Diet
Avoid any products containing wheat, rye and barley. Grains and starches such as rice, quinoa, millet and corn are all fine for the coeliac sufferer. Try lentil, corn or rice pasta. It's not uncommon for sufferers to be intolerant to other foods such as dairy products made from cow's milk. Try non-dairy soya or rice products instead. Often people who cannot tolerate cows' milk can try sheep's or goats' yoghurt with a little organic honey. Avoid foods containing refined sugar like shop-bought cakes and pre-packaged desserts. Lack of vitamin E has been linked to this problem, so eat

plenty of wheat germ, avocados and olive oil that are all rich in vitamin E.

Supplements

Glutenzyme, containing digestive enzymes which assist in the break down of gluten in the body. Liquid multi-vitamins are useful for this problem as they are easily absorbed through the gut wall. • [BC]

Quercetin Complex contains the powerful bioflavonoid quercetin, vitamin C and bromelain which aids digestion. Quercetin has a proven anti-histamine, anti-allergic activity. • [S]

The amino acid L glutamine helps to heal the lining of the digestive system. Essential fatty acids are vital for healing the gut lining (*see* **Fats You Need To Eat**). • [HN]

Reading

Diets to Help Gluten and Wheat Allergy by Rita Greer, £2.99. Thorsons.
Cooking Without, Barbara Cousins, £5.50. Available from 0171 436 5122.

Hints

Trufree Foods can supply a range of suitable flours for preparing a range of foods, plus dietary advice. Further information available from 0181 874 1130.

Research from Finland shows that small amounts (50–70g) of oat-based products can be tolerated by coeliacs without damaging intestinal absorption.

COLDS AND FLU

Colds and flu are caused by viruses. Flu symptoms generally are more severe and often include fever and aching. Because colds and flu are caused by viruses, antibiotics which are only effective against bacteria are of no use. When we are stressed or run down, our immune system works less efficiently and we become more prone to these infections.

Diet
Avoid all sugar, white flour and other refined carbo-hydrates because these can dampen the immune system. Cut out dairy products made from cows' milk which cause mucus formation, blocking sinuses and worsening the symptoms. Eat plenty of fresh fruit and vegetables. Drink at least six glasses of filtered water to help the body eliminate toxins (*see* **General Health Hints**).

Supplements
Take natural source beta-carotene complex to boost the immune system. Echinacea tablets or tincture helps drain the lymphatic system and fight viral infections. Vitamin C is a very potent anti-viral agent and can be very effective in reducing the severity and duration of an attack of cold or flu. At the onset of symptoms, take 1g of vitamin C straight away and keep repeating every two hours throughout the day until a day after the symptoms have gone.

Plus a liquid gel capsule multi-vitamin/mineral and a B complex. • **[FSC]**

Muccolyte, a complex containing vitamins A, C and D, potassium and digestive enzyme to support and maintain mucus membranes. Plus garlic capsules with main meals which really help to clear blocked sinuses. • **[BC]**

Hints
Wash your hands regularly if you are in contact with people who have a cold as viruses can easily permeate the soft skin on the palms of the hands. Viruses are airborne and spread quickly at large gatherings. Avoid being in stuffy, smoky

rooms for too long. Get plenty of exercise and fresh air.

Finely chop a 2½cm piece of fresh ginger, stand in boiling water for 15 minutes with lemon juice and freshly chopped spring onions; strain and sip.

Keep warm and avoid changes in the temperature of your surroundings for at least 48 hours until symptoms subside. Rest is essential if you have a temperature.

Reading
Colds and Flu by Penny Davenport, £3.99, Element Books.
Colds and Flu by Charles B Inlander and Cynthia K Moran, £3.99, Thorsons.

＊ ❋ ＊

COLD SORES

Cold sores are caused by the *herpes simplex* virus which once contracted, lies dormant in the body's nerves until it is activated again. The virus is more likely to become active by sudden exposure to hot or cold weather or sunlight. Another common trigger for cold sores is a weakened immune system. This is why cold sores are more likely to occur when we are stressed or run down.

Diet
Avoid nuts, chocolates and seeds for a month as they contain arginine, an amino acid on which the virus thrives. Eat plenty of wholegrain cereals, fish, fruit and vegetables which help resist infection. Avoid sugar and refined carbohydrates which tend to depress immune function. Some readers have found that dairy products made from cows' milk can trigger an attack. Use non-dairy soya or rice milk instead.

Supplements
By taking 1g of the amino acid lysine at the onset of symptoms, the attack is often stopped – because lysine interferes with replication of the herpes virus. One drop of liquid Bio-A daily in liquid (equivalent to 5,000iu of vitamin A) is an easily absorbed form of vitamin A. Histazyme, containing vitamin C, lysine, zinc, bromelain, vitamin A, manganese and B6, a natural anti-viral/inflammatory supplement. Plus 1g of vitamin C daily. Derma C cream applied topically at the first sign of any sores forming. • **[BC]**

Hints
Make sure you change your toothbrush regularly as this can carry the virus. Pierce a vitamin E capsule and apply directly onto the sores.

CONJUNCTIVITIS
Conjunctivitis is an inflammation of the outer surface of the eye and is often caused by allergies or viral and bacterial infections. If the condition is due to an allergy, the eyes are usually itchy and red but, other than tears, there is rarely a discharge. Other types of conjunctivitis are often accompanied by a thick mucus discharge and should be treated by your doctor. Most non-allergic cases of conjunctivitis will clear up on their own, but are usually helped by bathing the eyes in warm water.

Diet
Keep the diet clean and avoid sugar, dairy products and food additives, which can all make symptoms worse. Drink plenty of filtered or bottled water. Eat plenty of fresh fruits and vegetables which help to strengthen immune function and fight infection (*see* **General Health Hints**).

Supplements

Bilberry Ginkgo Eyebright Complex; bilberry improves overall eye function and, along with the herb ginkgo biloba, it benefits circulation and protects eyes from free radical damage. This formula also contains a nutritional anti-oxidant complex including carotenoids, vitamins A, C and E, and selenium. Echinacea, goldenseal and cat's claw complex contain powerful immune stimulating herbs which should help protect against infections of the eye – they are also anti-inflammatory. • [S]

Histazyme, containing calcium, vitamin C, zinc, B6, lysine and silica all to help heal tissue. NutriGuard Forte contains vitamins A, E and C plus natural carotenes, all anti-oxidants, which help support the immune system and the eyes. • [BC]

Hints

Conjunctivitis is highly contagious when caused by a viral infection. Use a Hi Tech Hygiene facial bath three times a day while infected, to clear and naturally disinfect the eyes, nose and nasal passages. Simply release a dropper of the liquid into a washbasin of warm/hot water with a dessertspoonful of salt dissolved in it. Lower your face into basin, holding your hair out of the way. Blink the eyes open and closed, and breathe out. Pat your face dry with a clean towel. Collodial silver, which kills some viruses and bacteria, can be safely dropped into the eyes with an eye dropper. It will not sting. For details, call 01435 882 880.

CONSTIPATION AND BLOATING (see also Flatulence)

The vast majority of cases of constipation are due to lifestyle and dietary factors. Lack of exercise is a common cause of constipation, as exercise stimulates the bowel to squeeze waste matter along it, rather like squeezing toothpaste from a tube. A diet that is low in fibre is another common cause. Although fibre is important for regular bowel function, fluid is essential too. Without enough fluid in the diet, fibre can get stuck in the gut, rather like cork in the neck of a wine bottle. Certain drugs including laxatives (which worsen constipation in the long term by allowing the bowel to become lazy), antibiotics and pain-killers all exacerbate constipation. A very common cause of bloating and wind is an overgrowth of candida or other unhealthy organisms in the gut (*see also* **Candida**). Here, the bloating and wind are caused by excessive quantities of gas, produced when candida ferments food. Food sensitivities (*see* **Allergies**) can also cause bloating.

Diet

Avoid bread and cereals containing wheat, as wheat bran often irritates the bowel making matters worse – oat bran and cereals are better. We all know that if you mix flour and water together it makes a glue-like paste and it does the same in the bowel! Melted cheese looks delicious but, once cold it sets like plastic; again this is what happens in the bowel, so also eliminate full-fat cheeses, especially when cooked. Avoid cows' milk products, use non-dairy soya or rice milk instead. Avoid beef and pork which are hard to digest and putrefy in a constipated gut. Treat yourself to a juicer and try a blend of organic cabbage, spinach, celery, apple, lemon juice and add one tablespoonful of organic extra virgin olive oil. Each day use a different blend of any fresh fruit or vegetables and drink these straight from the juicer whilst the enzymes are alive. Avoid too much tea and coffee, which dehydrate the bowel. Make sure you drink at least eight glasses of bottled or filtered water every day.

Supplements
Colon Care until normal movement is restored. Two Bio-Acidophilus taken daily to replace the good bacteria in the gut. (As antibiotics often cause constipation, these live bacteria are a must if you have taken antibiotics and are constipated as a result.) 200–400mg magnesium daily for one month which improves muscle movement within the bowel. • [BC]

If you are generally constipated, take a few chlorella or spirulina tablets daily which help to de-toxify the system. Raw organic linseeds are excellent for general health and to keep the bowel moving. Start with two teaspoons daily over cereal, gradually increasing to one tablespoon daily with plenty of water. Natural liquorice supplements are a good form of laxative.

Reading
Food Combining in 30 Days by Kathryn Marsden, £4.99, Thorsons.
Irritable Bowel Syndrome by Stephen Terrass, £4.99, Thorsons.

Hints
Aloe vera juice has been found helpful for many sufferers when four tablespoons are taken daily for several weeks.

Potter's make a Cleansing Herb Formula containing buckthorn bark, psyllium seeds and senna leaves. Available from good health stores.

Nature's Best make a supplement Ido-Air especially to help with bloating and flatulence, ask at your local health food store.

Walk briskly every day or take some other form of regular exercise (especially tummy exercise which helps to stimulate the bowel). When you feel the need to pass a motion, be sure not to ignore the signal; take the time to read a magazine on the loo! It really does help. Never bear down and strain excessively as this can increase your risk of developing piles and varicose veins.

For severe constipation especially after surgery – and with your doctor's permission – try colonic irrigation. I have a colonic two or three times a year as a thorough cleanse (*see* **Useful Information** *for further details*). You can also give yourself a home colonic. It help to re-educate the peristaltic movements and is called the Clysmatic, which is easy to use. For details, call 01435 882880.

COUGHS

Coughing can be due to infections such as colds and flu, asthma (especially if the coughing is at night), chest infections and smoking. Sometimes the cough may be accompanied by the production of phlegm. If this is yellow or green, it is a sign that you are suffering from a bacterial infection and you should see your doctor.

Diet
Avoid dairy products made from cow's milk which are well-known to increase mucus secretions and aggravate a cough. Also avoid sugar and refined carbohydrates which can suppress the immune system and reduce your body's ability to fight infection (*see* **General Health Hints**).

Supplements
Echinacea, goldenseal and cat's claw complex – all these herbs help to boost the immune system which helps protect against infections of the respiratory tract. • **[S]**

Buccalzyme, a formula containing zinc, echinacea and liquorice which enhances the immune system. Potassium ascorbate, a form of vitamin C with each meal, useful against viral infection. • **[BC]**

Hints

If you wheeze from time to time, it is possible that you may have asthma (*see* **Asthma**). Culpeper's Herbal Cough Mixture has given relief to many readers with chronic coughs. For further information call Culpeper's mail-order service on 01223 894054 or to find your nearest Culpeper store, call 01223 891196. Take two tablespoons of aloe vera juice every day to soothe your throat and boost your immune system. Zinc lozenges reduce severity and duration of cold symptoms and help relieve a tickly cough and throat.

CRAMPS

A painful muscular spasm or contraction, often caused by poor blood supply to the muscles. Many people think that cramps are caused by a salt deficiency but this is, in fact, quite rare. Cramp is more commonly caused by a lack of magnesium, calcium or potassium.

Diet

Potassium-rich foods such as fruit (especially bananas) and vegetables are recommended because potassium plays an important part in muscle contraction. If you exercise or sweat excessively you may be low in sodium. Rather than adding salt to your diet, go for naturally sodium-rich foods such as celery.

Green leafy vegetables, nuts and seeds, especially sesame seeds will give you much needed calcium and magnesium (*see* **General Health Hints**).

Supplements

Ginkgo Plus contains vitamin C as potassium ascorbate, ginkgo and the flavonoid bilberry, which are all known to

aid circulation. • [BC]

Super multi-mineral complex, containing calcium and magnesium which usually relieve cramp, plus 200iu of vitamin E to help improve blood flow to the muscles. • [FSC]

Hints
A regime of regular exercise is beneficial like walking, swimming or yoga. Regular massage of the feet and legs whilst raised will also help to improve circulation. See a chiropractor or try reflexology (*see* **Useful Information** *for further details*).

CROHN'S DISEASE
An inflammatory disease which can affect any part of the intestine. Common symptoms include abdominal pain, weight loss, loss of appetite, diarrhoea and fever. Because the bowel lining is diseased, its ability to absorb nutrients is often very limited leading to nutritional deficiencies, particularly in the mineral zinc.

Diet
Avoid foods known to cause bad reactions, the most common being dairy products made from cows' milk, wheat, oats, rye, barley, corn and any products which contain white flour and sugar. Artificial sweeteners containing fructose or sorbitol seem to be a problem for some sufferers. Consider food combining which improves digestion and absorption of food, and can help to take the stress off your digestive system.

Supplements
Gastroplex, a herbal compound containing slippery elm, marshmallow and gamma oryzanol to help soothe an

irritated stomach. Taken with each meal, this formula has been shown to aid digestion, together with liquid multivitamins which are more easily absorbed for people with disorders of the digestive tract. • **[BC]**

Take two acidophilus capsules to replace the good bacteria in the gut, along with a magnesium compound for cramps. B12 and bio-zinc, together with a calcium compound to help absorption of nutrients from food. • **[BLK]**

The amino acid glutamine taken daily helps to heal a leaky and inflamed gut, along with one tablespoon of Essential Balance Oil made from organic linseeds and pumpkin seeds which will help to heal the leaky gut. • **[HN]**

Reading
The Complete Guide to Digestive Health by K Mayes, £4.99, Thorsons.
How To Improve Digestion and Absorption by C Scarfe, £2.50, ION Press.

Hints
Crohn's Disease is exacerbated by stress, therefore any techniques known to reduce stress should prove helpful such as yoga, meditation, massage or hypnotherapy. Adequate rest is essential for any Crohn's sufferer and gentle exercise is also beneficial.

For further help, contact The National Association for Colitis and Crohn's Disease (NACC), 4 Beaumont House, Sutton Road, St Albans, Hertfordshire AL1 5HH.

Crohn's in Childhood Research Association (CICRA), Parkgate House, 356 West Barnes Lane, Motspur Park, Surrey KT3 6NB.

CYSTITIS

Cystitis is usually caused by a bacterial infection in the bladder. Symptoms include the urge to urinate and a burning sensation when passing water. Cystitis is more common in women than men. The cause of infection can often be confirmed by urine analysis, but regularly no bugs are found. In these cases the cause of the symptoms is often candida (*see* **Candida**) or food intolerance. **If symptoms are accompanied by fever and pain in one or both loins, this is a sign of kidney infection and you should consult your doctor immediately.**

Diet
Avoid products containing yeast and sugar like bread, cakes, biscuits and soft drinks. Also avoid vinegar, soy sauce, mushrooms and alcohol, which also contain yeast and sugar. Drink at least eight glasses of filtered or bottled water and eat a live organic low-fat yoghurt every day.

Supplements
UR228 Uritol Capsules and CP227 Cystoplex, made from cranberries which contain hippuric acid known to prevent bacteria clinging to the bladder wall. 2g of vitamin C with bioflavonoids, plus 200iu of vitamin E daily as an anti-inflammatory and to keep the bladder lining clean. Cervagyn cream can be applied topically to ease the itching.
• **[BC]**
   To lessen growth of yeast infections, take a yeast-free B complex with biotin and lactobacillus acidophilus capsules for at least six weeks. Cat's claw tea is helpful for urinary infections. Aloe Gold with 7% cranberry and cherry juice will help overcome infection and soothe the urinary passages. • **[HN]**

Reading
Bladder Problems by Rosy Reynolds, £3.99, Thorsons.

Cystitis: Prevention & Treatment by Angela Kilmartin, £4.99, Thorsons.

Cystitis Information Sheet. Send four first class stamps to Green Library, 9 Rickett Street, London SW6 1RU or call 0171 385 0012.

Hints
Drink plenty of water each day as this can help to flush out unhealthy organisms from the bladder. Urinate as soon as possible after having sexual intercourse to stop transmission of bugs into the bladder. If symptoms are acute, avoid intercourse for at least one week, as you can pass the bacteria from one partner to another. Avoid perfumed soaps and vaginal deodorants at all times, as chemicals are strongly implicated in this condition. Wear cotton underwear. Avoid tightly fitting jeans, especially in hot weather. Douche daily with diluted tea tree and lavender oil or add a few drops to your bath. Acupuncture and homeopathic remedies like cantharis have helped many sufferers (*see* **Useful Information** *for further details*).

DEPRESSION
Typical symptoms of depression are unhappiness, irritability, pessimism, fatigue, insomnia, headache, anxiety, loss of sex drive and feelings of negativity. It can also lead to loss of concentration and difficulty in making decisions. Poor eating habits can cause depression by failing to provide adequate nutrients for healthy brain function. Serotonin is the hormone in the brain which helps us to feel better. If we eat a junk diet, we may not produce enough serotonin which can lead to depression. You can also suffer depression if you are completely exhausted – get some rest! Some cases of depression are related to food intolerance

(*see* **Allergies**).

Diet

There is evidence that diets too high or too low in saturated fat can cause depression. Drinking more than four or five cups of coffee a day and eating too much refined sugar can also cause depression, as they deplete the body of vital nutrients like chromium, folic acid and vitamins C and B. Therefore, cut out caffeine and sugar from the diet. Eat a varied, wholefood diet rich in fruits and vegetables and low in saturated fat. Make sure that you eat the right kind of fats like virgin olive oil and oily fish which have an important role to play in healthy brain function (*see* **Fats You Need to Eat**). Investigate the possibility of a food intolerance as many people suffering from depression have an intolerance to wheat, eggs and cow's milk (*see* **General Health Hints**).

Supplements

50–75mg of B6 plus a B complex to support the nervous system.

500mg of niacinamide (vitamin B3) to help calm the nerves. Dr Abram Hoffer, a world expert in depression, treats most of his patients with large doses of niacinamide and vitamin C. He suggests 1g of B3, three times daily until the depression lifts. A multi-vitamin plus 2g of vitamin C and magnesium daily. • **[FSC]**

DLPA (an amino acid) has proved helpful as it lengthens the life of natural endorphins which are mood-enhancing substances made in the brain. • **[LGF]**

People with mild depression have reported significant improvement when taking the herb St John's Wort. Available in tablet and tinctures from good health stores.

Positive Nutrition is a specific formulation for depression containing the amino acids tyrosine and glutamine, plus the vitamins and minerals like B3, B6, magnesium and zinc needed to utilize the amino acids in the body. • **[HN]**

Lack of zinc is a common cause of depression, so take a multi-mineral containing zinc.

Reading
Overcoming Depression by Dr Caroline Shreeve, £5.99, Thorsons.
How to Stop Worrying and Start Living by Dale Carnegie, £5.99, Cedar.
Mental Health & Illness – The Nutrition Connection by Patrick Holford, £7.95, ION Press.
How To Heal Depression by Dr H Bloomfield, £7.99, Thorsons.
Stress, Anxiety and Insomnia by Michael Murray ND, £9.95, Prima Press. Available to order from 0171 436 5122.

Hints
Regular exercise stimulates the release of endorphins in the brain which have a mood-enhancing effect, increase blood flow to the brain and promote positive thinking. At least one study shows that aerobic exercise can be effective in reducing depression. Learn to breath properly by practising yoga. Visualization has been successful in relieving depression during clinical trials in America. Studies show that counselling and problem-solving sessions often prove more useful than anti-depressant drugs. Have a regular aromatherapy massage using oils like bergamot, geranium, lavender, rose, clary sage and sandalwood, which all help to lift one's spirits.

For details of a counsellor in your area, contact the British Association for Counselling (BAC), 1 Regent Place, Rugby CV21 2PJ. Tel: 01788 578328.

Many readers have found hypnotherapy very helpful for cases of chronic depression (*see* **Useful Information** *for further details*).

DIABETES

Diabetes Mellitus, or sugar diabetes as it is commonly known, is a condition in which the body's ability to handle sugar is impaired and blood sugar levels are higher than they should be. The condition comes in two main forms; juvenile onset and mature onset diabetes. Juvenile onset diabetes starts in childhood or adolescence and is due to a deficiency of the hormone insulin, which is responsible for keeping blood sugar levels in check. Juvenile onset diabetics accounts for about 10% of all diabetic cases. Mature onset diabetes usually starts in middle or old age and although adequate amounts of insulin are often produced, the body is resistant to its effects. Mature onset diabetes is very much associated with lifestyle factors such as being overweight, eating a diet high in sugar and refined carbohydrates, and taking too little exercise. Common symptoms of diabetes include fatigue, drowsiness, skin infections like boils, poor wound healing, thirst and frequent urination.

There are certain conditions which cannot be legally treated by alternative practitioners, and diabetes is one of them. The best course of action would be to ask your own GP to refer you to a nutritionist who is also a medical doctor, who can prescribe supplements and dietary changes to suit your needs (*see* **Useful Information** *for details*).

Diet

There are certain guidelines that may prove helpful with your doctor's approval. Avoid all foods and drinks containing sugar. Also avoid starches which release sugar quickly into the bloodstream including white bread, white rice and pasta made from refined flour. Eat foods which release sugar more slowly into the blood stream, such as wholegrain cereals like porridge, wholemeal bread, brown rice, wholewheat pasta and vegetables as lightly cooked as possible. Cut out alcohol, caffeine, chocolates, salt and saturated fats like those found in red meat and dairy products made from cows' milk. Replace full-fat milk with skimmed milk products or use soya milk which is non-dairy, low-fat and sugar-free. (Check labels carefully to make sure sugar-free is mentioned). Replace animal fats with mono-unsaturated fat such as extra virgin olive oil and use Vitaquell spread on your bread. Eat several evenly-spaced small meals daily to keep blood sugar levels regulated.

Supplements

B complex daily containing niacin and biotin. Chromium is helpful for controlling blood sugar levels, but should only be taken under medical supervision. Zinc is essential for insulin secretion. Also 1g of vitamin C with bioflavonoids, vitamin E 400iu (if you are low in natural vitamin E you are more likely to develop diabetes in later life). Fish oil capsules, garlic and lecithin granules, all taken daily have proved beneficial to some sufferers. • [LGF]

Reading

Victory Over Diabetes by Philpot and Kalita, £9.99, Keats. Available from ION, Tel: 0181 877 9993.
The Natural Way With Diabetes by Catherine Steven, £3.99, Element Books.
Diabetes and Hypoglycemia by Michael Murray NF, £9.95, Prima Press. Available to order from 0171 436 5122.

Hints

Always let practitioners know you are diabetic. Regular eye checks and foot care are also recommended as both can be affected in diabetes. Bilberry extract is useful for preventing onset of diabetic cataracts.

Diacur, a combination of homeopathic remedies from France has been used successfully in the management of diabetes and is now available in the UK. For details, call 01435 882880.

Many people who have diabetic problems suffer with

poor circulation in their feet. Reflexology has proved very helpful for circulation (*see* **Useful Information** *for further details*). Alternatively, you could try an energy roller which works on the same principle as reflexology – roll bare feet for two minutes daily on the roller; this hurts initially but it gets easier! For further details, send an SAE to Shakti Chakra, PO Box 3984, London SE12 0EJ. Regular exercise is vital when treating diabetes as it can reduce the need for insulin. Try walking for at least 15 minutes, increasing to 30 minutes daily or more. Hypolarm is a perspiration alarm which has a sensor that attaches to the skin. The alarm is used while asleep and a two tone alarm wakes the user to warn of a dangerously low fall in sugar levels. For further information, contact 0181 441 9641.

DIARRHOEA

Causes include infection with a bacterium, virus or parasite, food poisoning, food allergy or intolerance and yeast overgrowth. Less frequently, diarrhoea can be caused by more severe conditions which affect the bowel such as ulcerative colitis and Crohn's disease. Diarrhoea is usually a short-term problem which will get better on its own. **If it is persistent, it is important to see your doctor.**

Diet

Make sure you drink plenty of fluids during an attack and for at least one day after it has stopped, to prevent dehydration which can make you feel dreadful. The best fluids are filtered water and diluted fresh vegetable juices. The diet should be kept as light as possible, so that the digestive tract gets a chance to rest. Fresh vegetable soups are usually well-tolerated, moving on to more solid food only when your symptoms seem much better.

Supplements
Goldenseal capsules (the herb goldenseal is known to kill most harmful organisms which typically cause diarrhoea). Multi-acidophilus powder (acidophilus, bifidobacterium and bulgaricus) to replenish the healthy bacteria in the gut. • [S]

Lack of zinc is often linked to diarrhoea. Take 30mg of elemental zinc daily whilst attack lasts and take a multi-mineral containing zinc thereafter.

Reading
How To Improve your Digestion and Absorption by Christopher Scarfe, £2.50, ION.

Hints
If travelling abroad, take acidophilus capsules for at least one week prior to travel and throughout your holiday. This keeps the level of healthy bacteria in the gut high which can help to keep bad bugs at bay. Bee Propolis is a natural antibiotic, as is grapefruit seed extract. Potter's make a Spanish Tummy Mixture containing herbs and tinctures to heal the gut. Available from all good health stores.

Never drink tap water unless you are sure it is safe to do so and avoid salads washed in local tap water. Eat only thoroughly cooked foods if you are worried about getting a bad tummy upset. Use bottled water and fizzy drinks but **only** if they have sealed tops and have not been previously tampered with.

DIVERTICULAR DISEASE or Diverticulitis
As we age, we can develop little pouches in the lining of the large intestine called *diverticulae*. This condition affects the

descending colon which is situated on the left hand side of the abdomen. Therefore any pain from diverticultis is usually felt on the left-hand side. This is more likely to happen if our diet is low in fibre. Chronic constipation is the most common underlying cause of this condition (*see* **Constipation**). Generally, these little pockets do not cause any problems but if one or more of them should become infected, it is possible to suffer from bleeding, diarrhoea, abdominal pain and fever. **Occasionally a pouch may burst; this is a serious condition requiring emergency medical attention.**

Diet

Fibre is important for managing this disorder but while the bowel is inflamed, avoid abrasive fibre like wheat bran. Initially, try soothing foods such as lightly stewed organic apples, creamed oats made with non-dairy soya milk along with soya yoghurts and ice cream. Avoid all foods containing pips and seeds which may lodge in the pouches. Take two tablespoons of aloe vera juice daily to help heal the lining of the gut. Stop eating refined foods such as white bread, cakes, biscuits, take-aways and pre-packaged meals which are full of additives, salt and sugar. Avoid red meats and all saturated fats.

Once the inflammation settles, try a little vegetable soup, steamed or grilled fish, or skinless poultry. Eat lots of garlic (or take garlic capsules) which helps combat infection. Eat live, low-fat yoghurt every day. Gradually increase your intake of fibre-rich foods like vegetables, brown rice, brown bread, millet, pulses, oat-based cereals and fruit. Drink at least eight glasses of filtered water each day. Use extra virgin olive oil for your salad dressing. Avoid meat and all yeast-based foods like Marmite, Bovril, cheese, soy sauce and mushrooms. Concentrated sweeteners that contain fructose and sorbitol may need to be eliminated as both have been found to cause a range of digestive problems in certain people. Carageenan is a milk protein stabilizer, often used in ice cream, that creates a problem for many sufferers.

Supplements
Pure Slippery Elm soothes sensitive digestive tracts. Chew 2–3 tablets before meals with a large glass of water. • **[BLK]**

Essential fatty acids, like GLA (gamma linolenic acid) and healthy bacteria such as acidophilus are vital for healing the gut lining. • **[NC]**

Take liquid gel multi-vitamins which are easily absorbed, plus 2mg of folic acid and 10,000iu of vitamin A daily to help healing of damaged tissue. • **[FSC]**

Reading
The Irritable Bowel Diet Book by Rosemary Nicol, £5.99, Sheldon Press.
Irritable Bowel Syndrome by Nigel Howard, £3.99, Element Books.
Irritable Bowel and Diverticulosis by Shirley Trickett, £5.99, Thorsons.
Beat IBS Through Diet by Maryon Stewart & Dr Alan Stewart, £8.99, Vermilion.

DIZZY SPELLS (*see* **Low Blood Sugar, Low Blood Pressure** *and* **Vertigo**)

EARACHE (*see also* **Tinnitus** *and* **Vertigo**)
Most earaches are caused by the build-up of fluid in the middle ear which can lead to an infection causing pain,

fever and loss of hearing. Children under the age of five are particularly prone to earache, often caused by sensitivity to foods such as corn, peanuts, cows' milk and wheat. Cows' milk products are very often the culprit. If you are able to identify the problem foods and eliminate them from the diet, the ear problems usually clear up.

Diet
Try replacing cows' milk with goats' or rice milk products which can be found in good health stores. Avoid refined foods, especially sugary or salty items. Eat a good balanced wholefood diet high in fresh salads, fruits and vegetables (*see* **General Health Hints**).

Supplements
The continuous use of antibiotics destroy not only the unhealthy bacteria responsible for the ear infection, but also the good bacteria in the gut which help digestion and support the immune system. To replace the good bacteria, add a quarter of a teaspoon of acidobifidus powder to food or drink daily for four weeks. From then on, include a live low-fat yoghurt every day (if your child is not sensitive to dairy products) or continue with the powder three times a week. Powder must be kept in the fridge to keep the bacteria alive.

A natural alternative to antibiotics, which does not destroy the good bacteria in the gut, is a liquid extract from grapefruit seed called Citricidal. Use 2–5 drops twice daily in juice to help the child through the infection and a few drops can be diluted and placed on cotton wool in the ear. • **[HN]**

An excellent hypo-allergenic, chewable multi-vitamin for children is Animal Fun by Natural Flow, together with zinc and evening primrose oil. • **[LGF]**

Hints

For irritations in the ears and sinuses, mucus and catarrh, use ear candles which gently and effectively remove excess ear wax without pain. Excellent for children. For details, call 0171 976 6615.

Do not let a child swim underwater if their ears become infected.

For a free Allergy Factsheet and details of an allergy blood test, send a large SAE to: Higher Nature, The Nutrition Centre, Burwash Common, East Sussex TN19 7LX.

See a cranial osteopath or chiropractor to check the alignment of the head and neck, as misalignment can cause earache (*see* **Useful Information** *for details*).

ECZEMA

Many readers have written to me about this very distressing complaint, which is an inflammatory disorder of the skin. Sometimes eczema is triggered by an external irritant, but often the condition is due to a reaction to something in the diet. Eczema can affect us at any point in our lives and tends to vary in severity from time to time. It is always worse when the body is under stress or exhausted, so make time for yourself and learn to relax with yoga or meditation. Non-steroidal anti-inflammatory drugs like Ibuprofen have been known to trigger an attack in some people.

Diet

Keep to a diet full of fresh salads, fruits and vegetables, (organic when possible), as it is necessary to avoid all food additives, pesticides, colourings and refined foods generally. Most common food sensitivities are due to dairy products made from cows' milk, peanuts, potatoes, eggs, red meat and some types of fish (*see* **Allergies**). Drink at least six glasses of filtered water daily. Healthy essential fats can help dampen down the inflammation, therefore include oily fish and sunflower, pumpkin and linseeds in your daily diet, along with avocados which are rich in mono-unsaturated fats and vitamin E. Seeds also contain zinc which is vital for skin healing. Buy organic seeds from the health store which have no additives or colourings and eat foods rich in magnesium like apricots, pears, peaches, fresh sweetcorn and green leafy vegetables.

Supplements
Essential Balance Oil made from organic cold pressed linseeds, pumpkin and sunflower seeds. An adult should take one tablespoon daily in juice and a child one teaspoon. This oil helps to heal a leaky gut which is often associated with eczema and helps to heal the skin. It needs to be kept in the fridge and never heated. • **[HN]**

1g of vitamin C with bioflavonoids daily which have a natural anti-inflammatory effect. Children's B-complex (as these are more easily absorbed). One drop of liquid vitamin A plus a liquid multi-vitamin in juice to help the skin. • **[NC]**

Zinc 30–60mg, essential for healing. Take daily until condition improves. Digestive enzymes may be particularly helpful as incomplete digestion of foods can lead to allergic reactions. **(Not to be taken by people who have stomach ulcers.)** • **[LGF]**

Reading
Super Skin by Kathryn Marsden, £5.99, Thorsons.
Eczema & Psoriasis by Stephen Terrass, £4.99, Thorsons.

Hints
Many readers have found that aloe vera taken internally and used topically has been helpful for eczema.

Mr Donald Walsh, DHM, MSHI, founded the Cherryfield

Clinic in 1986. His herbal preparations, which are taken internally and used externally, have proved extremely successful in treating skin conditions. For further details, contact the Hale Clinic on 0171 631 0156.

If an allergy to some food is suspected, then avoid the offending food (*see* **Allergies**). Avoid soaps and soap powders; use soap substitutes or Dead Sea soaps available from good pharmacies and health stores.

Chinese herbs have proved exceptionally helpful in many cases but you need to see a qualified Chinese herbalist and may need to have liver function checked before and during treatment. Others report great success through homeopathy (*see* **Useful Information** *for further details*).

For further help, contact The National Eczema Society, 4 Tavistock Place, London WC1H 9RA.

ELECTRICAL STRESS

Every cell in the human body has its own electro-magnetic field which is affected by all the electrical equipment around us in everyday life. 60 years ago hardly any household owned a radio, never mind a television, computer, microwave, mobile phone or electric blanket. In a very short space of time we have made a world in which we are being bombarded by a dangerous enemy. Electrical pollution is thought to be one of the fastest growing causes of many major diseases. It took scientists 30 years to discover that excessive exposure to X-ray machines could cause cancer, and only recently have they started to realize how long-term exposure to electricity can affect the human body.

People who live near power lines and sub-stations and whose homes are full of electrical equipment, seem to be more prone to illnesses like ME (chronic fatigue), cancers, migraines and insomnia. Research has also shown that if there is subterranean water under a home, then this can also compound the problems because water can transmit electrical energy. Night and day, these electromagnetic rays pass through the delicate cells of our bodies, which were not designed to withstand such influences.

Electrical pollution can affect just about any component of your health. For instance, every time you turn on a light switch, your brain's rhythms immediately change. Spending too much time under fluorescent lighting or in front of a computer screen can suppress the brain chemical melatonin. This can have effects as diverse as infertility, insomnia and depression. Recent research from the National Council on Radiation Protection, which advises the American government, stated that even common household appliances, such as food mixers and vacuum cleaners, send out enough electromagnetic radiation to cause heart disease, Parkinson's and Alzheimer's by suppressing production of melatonin in the pineal gland in the brain.

Reading
Something In The Air by Roger Coghill, £12.99. Available to order from Coghill Research on 01495 763389. Well worth reading for anyone who wants to know more about this subject.

Hints
Keep electrical appliances in the bedroom to a minimum. Turn off all mains switches in the bedroom at night. If you live near an electrical power station, put large copper jugs or ornaments in the windows. Avoid using electric blankets. Always stand at least three feet away from a microwave when it's working. (Studies show that microwaving can alter the chemistry of food.) Irradiating (X-raying) food could, in the long run, prove very dangerous. If any food like strawberries are still healthy looking after being in

your fridge for a few days, then they have most likely been irradiated.

The Harmony Balance Centre sell Transend Cards on which are imprinted holograms programmed to enhance the energy of the body and give some protection from electrical stress. They also supply bottles of special crystals which harmonize the environment and protect against electrical and geopathic stresses (radiation which comes up from faults underground). For further details of the cards and harmony bottles, send a large SAE to Jacqui Beacon, The Harmony Balance Centre, PO Box 3912, London NW11 6AZ.

There is a BioElectric Shield pendant made from sterling silver which contains a matrix of quartz and other crystals. It has been scientifically designed to reflect and re-direct electromagnetic radiation from computers, TVs, mobile phones etc. Double-blind trials have shown that, by wearing the shield many conditions associated with environmental and electrical stress are relieved. Costs £110. For details, call 0181 640 2095.

The Coghill Research Laboratories have invented a small, easy to use, instrument called The Coghill Fieldmouse (£58.75), which tells you if you are in a high electrical energy atmosphere. For details, send a large SAE to: Coghill Research, Lower Race, Pontypool, Gwent NP4 5UF.

Have your home dowsed by an expert if you are worried about suffering from over-exposure from electricity. Send an SAE to: The British Society of Dowsers, Sycamore Barn, Tamley Lane, Hastingleigh, Ashford, Kent TN25 5HW. Tel: 01233 750253.

EMPHYSEMA
Emphysema is a condition of middle and old age which affects the lungs, resulting in a reduced capacity to absorb

oxygen and difficulty in expelling air. Sufferers usually complain of increasing breathlessness made worse by exercise. Almost always, emphysema is caused by long-term smoking or from inhaling chemical gases.

Diet
Eat a healthy diet based on wholegrains, fruits and vegetables. Nutritional deficiencies are common and a healthy diet can help to provide the nutrients that help the body use oxygen (*see* **General Health Hints**). If there is a lot of phlegm associated with the coughing, it is possible that there is an underlying food intolerance. If this is the case, try eliminating dairy products made from cows' milk for two weeks to see whether symptoms improve (*see* **Allergies**).

Supplements
NutriGuard (an antioxidant containing high potency lycopene and other natural carotenes, which helps protect the integrity of the mucous membranes and improves resistance to infections).

2g of vitamin C to aid healing and increase immune resistance against infections. 100iu of vitamin E with each meal which helps the body utilize oxygen. • **[BC]**

Cat's Claw Tea, a powerful immune stimulant to help clear the lungs. Aloe Gold Juice – take daily to boost immunity and help repair lung tissue. • **[HN]**

Reading
Asthma and Bronchitis by Jan de Vries, £4.99, Mainstream Publishing.

Hints
Santaherba – a French homeopathic remedy which helps to ease mucus congestion. • **[NC]**

Gentle exercise can help relieve the symptoms of this condition, especially regular walking, swimming or cycling.

Start slowly and build up gradually. Reflexology has proved successful with some sufferers. Yoga can also be beneficial as this therapy will teach you relaxation techniques and how to breathe properly (*see* **Useful Information** *for further details*).

Aromatherapy has also been of benefit to some sufferers. Fill a basin with boiling water and add three drops of oil of eucalyptus aromatherapy oil. Put your head over the basin with a towel over you to trap the steam and inhale deeply for two to five minutes, keeping your eyes closed.

ENDOMETRIOSIS

Endometriosis is a condition where tissue, which normally lines the womb, is found outside the womb, in places such as the ovaries, the fallopian tubes or the pelvis. No one knows what causes the condition, but there is a theory that during menstruation, womb tissue flows not only down to the vagina, but up through the fallopian tubes, eventually sticking to other structures. The most common symptoms of endometriosis are pain at the time of ovulation, painful periods and pain on sexual intercourse. Endometriosis is also a common cause of infertility.

Some nutritional doctors believe there is a significant link between endometriosis and candida overgrowth in the gut or vagina. Many women have symptoms which are assumed to be due to endometriosis which disappear or are significantly relieved when they are treated for candida. There is also evidence linking the chemical dioxin used in the production process of making sanitary products to this condition. Always use pure cotton tampons.

Diet
If you suspect candida (tell-tale symptoms include thrush,

abdominal bloating and wind, food cravings and fatigue), then you should avoid sugar, refined carbohydrates and yeast (*see* **Candida**). As a general rule, avoid alcohol, sugar and processed foods which may have a lot of synthetic additives. Food sensitivities may make endometriosis worse, so it may well be worth you having these allergies investigated.

Supplements
Dysmenorrhoea (painful, heavy periods) are a classic feature in those with endometriosis. The omega 6 fatty acid GLA (gamma linolenic acid) has been shown to be helpful in relieving dysmenorrhoea. Both EPA (an omega 3 fatty acid) and GLA also possess anti-inflammatory activity (*for further details, see* **Fats You Need to Eat**).

Free radical damage may be a major contributing factor in alterations in uterine tissue and various hormonal dysfunctions. Anti-oxidant nutrients, especially vitamin E, selenium, vitamin C and carotenoids may be very helpful in preventing or helping relieve disturbances of the reproductive system, as well as strengthening connective tissue in the uterus. Therefore, take an anti-oxidant formula daily. Genistein Soy Isoflavone Extract, as excessive oestrogen is linked to endometriosis, so the blocking of excessive levels with genistein may be extremely beneficial. Genistein is also a very powerful anti-oxidant. Various B vitamins, especially B6 and folic acid may be helpful in endometriosis. 500mg of L-Methionine, this amino acid is known to help detoxify oestrogen in the liver. • **[S]**

Reading
Balancing Hormones Naturally by Kate Neil, £4.95, ION Press. Available from 0181 877 9993.

Hints
Homeopathy has proved beneficial to many sufferers as has

Chinese medicine (*see* **Useful Information** *for further details*).

Further help is available from the National Endometriosis Society, Suite 59 Westminster Palace Gardens, 1–7 Artillery Row, London SW1P 1RL or call 0171 222 2776.

You may also find a chat with the Women's Nutritional Advisory Service on 01273 487366 helpful.

EXHAUSTION (*see also* **ME** *and* **Stress**)

When we are exhausted, it seems that there is no escape from the daily spiral of stress which makes us feel worse. In order to escape from this dilemma, it is essential to have a complete rest. One good night's sleep and a few extra vitamins are not sufficient help once the body is totally exhausted. If at all possible take a few days off and have a complete rest. Total exhaustion is cumulative and the immune system becomes less and less effective, until you get sick or stressed out and **have** to stop. Take at least one hour every day to call your own. Try meditating (*see* **Meditation**) or have a warm bath with a few added drops of lavender oil. Go for a leisurely walk. If you find it hard to sleep because you are over-tired, then try to set aside one morning a week when you can have a lie-in to help re-charge your batteries instead of laying awake worrying about getting no sleep! (*see* **Insomnia**). Low blood sugar is a common cause of fluctuating energy levels and food cravings (*see* **Low Blood Sugar**).

Diet

Avoid stimulants like coffee, tea, cola, sugar and chocolate. Sugar-based junk foods lower the immune system and can disrupt blood sugar levels. Keep to a healthy diet which includes plenty of live food like fruit, vegetables and alfalfa which give you more energy. Refuse to eat late at night, especially heavy rich foods like red meat and protein which take a long time to digest. You are better off eating complex carbohydrates at night such as vegetables and wholegrains as these have a more calming effect (*see* **General Health Hints**).

Supplements
An anti-oxidant multi-vitamin formula, 50mg of CoEnzyme Q10, is known to help boost energy levels when taken regularly. Call PharmaNord for details on 0800 591756.

2g of vitamin C daily can help boost the immune system.

Take Pantothenic acid (B5) 500–1,000mg plus a B complex for six weeks to support the adrenal and nervous system which is under stress when we are exhausted. 1g of Siberian ginseng, known as an energy booster (not to be taken if you suffer from high blood pressure). Stress lowers magnesium levels, take 200–600mg a day. • **[FSC]**

Reading
All Day Energy by Kathryn Marsden, £4.99, Bantam Books.
Energise Yourself by Vera Peiffer, £5.99, Thorsons.
Tired All The Time by Dr Alan Stewart, £7.99, Optima.

Hints
Gentle exercise like yoga, Tai Chi or Qigong helps to make you feel more positive and re-build energy levels.

Blue-green algae, chlorella and spirulina are also known to help raise energy levels and reduce feelings of exhaustion. For details, call 0181 390 9362.

If at all practical treat yourself to three days at a health spa to rejuvenate and rest.

EYE PROBLEMS (*see also* **Cataracts**)

I have received thousands of letters about various eye conditions – the most common are included here. Many elderly people suffer from eye problems which can be associated with poor circulation. Problems with circulation are particularly important when they affect the seeing part of the eye called the retina. Supplements necessary for healthy eyes are vitamin C, natural source beta-carotene, vitamin E, bilberry, zinc and selenium. Individuals with brown eyes often have problems with metabolizing fats so if you have brown eyes, watch your saturated fat intake. Blue-eyed people tend to suffer more acid conditions like arthritis, ulcers and asthma. Green-eyed individuals have a tendency to liver and digestive problems.

EYE PROBLEMS – BLEPHARITIS

A condition where calcium deposits lodge under the eyelids especially at the edges causing redness and irritation.

Diet

Eat more green vegetables and citrus fruits. Avoid red meats, cheese, spinach, chocolate, sugar and animal fats. Bioflavonoid-rich foods like bilberries, blueberries and cherries are known to help soothe the eyes.

Supplements

One Mega GLA (gamma linolenic acid), an essential fatty acid which has an anti-inflammatory effect. Procydin, contains bilberry, black cherry and blackberry extracts which are high in bioflavonoids known to support delicate eye tissue. NutriGuard Forte, containing natural beta-carotene, selenium and vitamins E, C and A. Bio-magnesium, as magnesium helps keep calcium in suspension which may stop the deposits forming. • **[BC]**

A compress made with cucumber helps to reduce inflammation. Drink rosehip tea daily which contains bioflavonoids and vitamin C.

Hints
Mix one teaspoonful of bicarbonate of soda with one pint of boiled water. Allow to cool, then apply gently to the blisters inside your eyelid with a cotton bud.

EYE PROBLEMS – ITCHY EYES
Itching in the eyes can be due to an infection like conjunctivitis, allergies like hayfever or exposure to a smoky or polluted atmosphere. Dry, itchy red eyes can also be caused by extreme tiredness. Get some sleep! Anyone with difficulty focusing should have their eyes tested and eye pain or discomfort should always be referred to a doctor.

Diet
Eat plenty of green vegetables and fresh produce in your diet, especially broccoli and carrots, organic whenever possible, that are rich in natural beta-carotene to help the eyes (*see* **General Health Hints**).

Supplements
Dry eyes and tear ducts can sometimes be a symptom of a lack of vitamins A, C and E. Take 2g of vitamin C daily plus a multi-vitamin or a specific formula such as Cantassium's Ocutrien or Se-Power. • **[LGF]**

Bilberry extract is an excellent herb used to treat poor vision, cataracts and support eye tissue. B vitamins, especially B2, can be effective in relieving dry eyes. • **[S]**

Hints

Eyebright herb can be made into a tea and when, cooled, used as an eye lotion or in tablet form from Natural Flow as Eyebright Extra. It has anti-inflammatory, astringent and anti-catarrhal properties. The homeopathic version of eyebright, *euphrasia*, can be used for bathing the eyes and is very soothing. Use Euphrasia Mother Tincture about four times a day using a disposable eye bath. Most good health stores should be able to order this, or call 0181 874 1130.

Don't use anyone else's face cloth or towel just in case the problem is infectious. If your eyes are inflamed, chloride compound is useful to reduce redness around the eyes. For details, call 0181 987 8640. Camomile tea is very soothing and helps reduce redness. Make an infusion with the tea bags. When cooled, place on the eyes for fifteen minutes.

EYE PROBLEMS – OPTIC NEURITIS

This is an inflammation of the optic nerve which carries information from the seeing part of the eye, the retina, to the brain. It can cause partial or complete loss of vision which comes on over a few hours or days and may be accompanied by a pain in the eye. Optic neuritis can sometimes be one of the symptoms of multiple sclerosis.

Diet

Try cutting out alcohol and caffeine which can interfere with blood circulation to the eye (*see* **General Health Hints**).

Supplements

Bioflavonoids with gingko biloba are known to improve the integrity of the blood capillaries and strengthen the tissues of the eyes. Liquid vitamin A is helpful for eye problems, one drop daily in juice. NutriGuard Forte contains beta-carotene, selenium and vitamins E, A and C. Vitamin B helps to support nerves in the eye area; take a B complex. • **[BC]**

EYE PROBLEMS – PUFFY EYES

A common cause of this problem is an allergic reaction, either to something you are eating regularly, or to an external allergen like the house dust mite, spray perfumes, paint, etc. See a kinesiologist who can determine the exact causes of the allergy which you can then avoid, or have an allergy test (*see* **Useful Information**). It can also be a sign of poor lymph circulation or kidney weakness (*see* **Allergies**).

Diet
Avoid salt in the diet as this will worsen any existing water retention. Also avoid tea, coffee, colas and all pre-packaged foods which often have a high salt, sugar and additive content. The most likely food allergens are wheat and products made from cows' milk. Cut these foods out of the diet for a couple of weeks to see if it helps. Drink at least six glasses of filtered water each day as not drinking enough can encourage the body to retain fluid.

Supplements
Digestive Enzyme supplements with HCl (Hydrochloric Acid) taken with each main meal may be helpful if problems are food related. (Do not take HCl if you have stomach ulcers or inflammation in the stomach.) A multi-vitamin tablet, two celery seed extract and 1g of vitamin C as potassium ascorbate help drainage. • **[BC]**

Hints
Manual Lymph Drainage (MLD) can also aid this condition

(*see* **Useful Information** *for further details*). A herbal supplement like Lymph Herba is also useful for relieving congestion in the lymphatic system. For details, call 0171 436 5122.

Make an infusion with camomile tea bags and, when cool, apply to the eyes.

Bach flower remedies have been found very useful for this condition as has reflexology (*see* **Useful Information** *for further details*).

Some readers report that their puffy eyes were related to an underactive thyroid, therefore if the problem is persistent, have a thorough check-up with your GP.

EYE PROBLEMS – RED-RIMMED EYES

Persistently red-rimmed eyes can be a sign of malnutrition and lack of vitamin B. It can also be a sign that your body is not absorbing all the nutrients it needs from your diet due to poor digestion.

Diet
Drink plenty of filtered water and keep your diet clean (*see* **General Health Hints**).

Supplements
Take a vitamin B supplement daily, along with a multi-vitamin and a digestive enzyme with all main meals, which will aid absorption of vital nutrients. If your eyes are inflamed, take an anti-inflammatory mineral supplement like chloride compound which helps reduce redness. • **[BLK]**

Hints
Bathe the eyes in cooled camomile tea which is very

soothing. Red-rimmed eyes can also indicate toxicity or allergies. Try Herbal Clear containing dandelion, burdock, milk thistle, vitamin C and niacin to detoxify the liver. • [HN]

Reading for general eye problems
The Bates Method by Peter Mansfield, £6.99, Vermilion.
Seeing Without Glasses by Robert-Michael Caplan, £12.30. Available from 0171 436 5122.

General hints for eye problems
Trayner Pinhole Glasses help strengthen weak eye muscles. For further details write to Trayner Pinhole Glasses, Upton Noble, Shepton Mallet, Somerset BA4 6BB or call 01749 850822.

FATIGUE (*see also* **Exhaustion** *and* **Stress**)

FATS YOU NEED TO EAT

It is important to minimize consumption of saturated animal fats, but cutting out too much fat from the diet can deprive us of essential fats which play a vital role in keeping us healthy. According to Dr Udo Erasmus, the world's leading authority on fats and oils, 'If you have dry skin, water retention, increased thirst, physical and mental exhaustion, emotional imbalance and inflammatory diseases like eczema and arthritis; or frequent infections, allergies, behavioural problems or cardiovascular disease, these are the first signs of essential fat deficiency'. A deficiency in these fats is also linked to such problems as high blood pressure, dry eyes and poor memory.

117

Diet

There are two types of essential fatty acids (EFAs: omega 6 and omega 3). They are termed essential because the body needs them but cannot manufacture them itself. Omega 3 fats are most commonly found in oily fish like mackerel and salmon and linseeds. Omega 6 fats are found in evening primrose oil, starflower oil, walnut and sesame oil. EFAs aid proper brain function, co-ordination and mood as well having a regulatory effect on the level of cholesterol in the blood. They also maintain water balance in the body and decrease inflammatory conditions like arthritis. Linseed oil, also known as flaxseed oil, contains both omega 3 and omega 6 in the correct balance. Sprinkle one tablespoon of linseeds onto breakfast cereal daily and mix the oil with olive oil for salad dressings.

Supplements

Take one tablespoon of Essential Balance oil made from cold pressed organic linseeds, pumpkin and sunflower seeds which has the correct ratio of omega 3 and 6 for better health. From all good health stores or call 01435 882880. Dr Erasmus has developed an oil called Udo's Choice made from organic flax seed, sunflower and sesame seed oils which, again, has a perfect balance of omega 3 and 6 essential fats. From all good health stores or call 0171 436 5122 or 0113 230 1993. These oils are highly unstable and should always be kept in the fridge and never heated. Add one tablespoon cold to any juice or salad dressings every day for improved skin, digestion and circulation.

Reading

The Fats We Need to Eat by Jeannette Ewin, £6.99, Thorsons.
The Fats That Heal and Fats That Kill by Udo Erasmus, £14.50, Alive Books. This book explains exactly what happens when we eat bad fats and dispels many myths about 'healthy' fats. Although a few chapters are a little technical,

skip these and just read the facts. A brilliant book for doctors. To order call 0181 877 9993.

Hints
I always take this oil in freshly-made juice each day. If you don't like this idea then take a 1g linseed oil capsule daily. Avoid buying refined oils from supermarkets and never fry food as this makes the fat rancid, which can cause cancer. Any oils or fats that have been hydrogenated or have trans-fats on the label are to be avoided at all costs. Include more virgin olive oil in your diet and eat these oils cold in salad dressings.

FIBROIDS
A fibroid is a benign tumour made up of muscle and fibrous tissue which grows in the muscular wall of the womb. Fibroids often produce no symptoms at all, but they are known to cause heavy menstrual bleeding and may occasionally contribute to infertility. The growth of fibroids seems to be related to a hormone imbalance, especially an excess of the hormone oestrogen. If you are on the combined Pill or HRT, both of which contain oestrogen, you may wish to discuss coming off these drugs with your GP, in order to help prevent further growth. Always consult a doctor if you have very heavy periods.

Diet
There are certain foods which contain plant substances similar to oestrogen that can actually help to lower oestrogen activity levels. The most potent being broccoli and soya products, as well as cabbage, Brussels sprouts and cauliflower. Eat these vegetables raw to maximize their effect or make fresh vegetable juice daily and drink immedi-

ately. Regular intake of raw organic linseeds (like Linusit Gold from health food stores), contains a substance called lignin which also helps to balance hormone levels. Reduce all animal fats and increase your intake of fibre which helps to reduce the production of oestrogen (*see* **General Health Hints**).

Supplements
Start taking 1g of vitamin C with bioflavonoids daily, along with 200iu of vitamin E and a multi-vitamin. The herbs dong quai and agnus castus are well known for their balancing effects on hormones. • **[LGF]**

There is also evidence to show that a regular intake of natural beta-carotene can help this condition.

It has been shown that many women do not ovulate after the age of thirty-five and therefore no longer make progesterone but still make oestrogen. Talk to your doctor about trying natural progesterone, which can help reverse or hold fibroids in check. For further information, send £2 to: The Natural Progesterone Information Service, BCM 4315, London WC1N 3XX.

Reading
Balancing Hormones Naturally by Kate Neil, £4.95, ION Press.

Hints
Once you reach your menopause, fibroids should shrink quite naturally.

FLATULENCE (*see also* **Constipation and Bloating**)
Very often bloating and wind are due to an imbalance in the organisms in the gut which can lead to excessive fermentation and therefore wind. It is almost always a

prominent feature of candida in the gut (*see* **Candida**). Poor digestion is another common cause of flatulence because undigested food makes a hearty meal for any unhealthy organisms that may be lurking in the gut. Other common causes of flatulence include swallowing air and the consumption of fizzy drinks and fermentable carbohydrates such as beans.

Diet
Certain foods especially pulses, beans, cabbage, Jerusalem artichokes, onions and garlic can cause flatulence in some people. Chewing foods well and not hurrying meals or eating excessively at any one meal will help. Food combining is known to help alleviate this problem by allowing more complete digestion of food. If you eat pulses, soak them overnight and discard the water; then boil them in fresh water along with a strip of kombu seaweed; this can help to reduce flatulence by breaking down the enzymes in the beans. Include fresh ginger in your diet which stimulates gastric juices and aids proper digestion. Eat more low-fat live yoghurt (*see* **General Health Hints**).

Supplements
Alphazyme, a digestive enzyme taken with main meals, which helps to digest plant carbohydrates (a common cause of fermentation and wind). For three months, take bio-acidophilus twice daily to replenish good bacteria in the gut, which also aids digestion. • [BC]

Hints
Chronic flatulence can also be a symptom of food intolerance, irritable bowel syndrome, candida or gut infections. If you are concerned, see a qualified nutritionist (*see* **Useful Information** *for details*).

FLU (*see* **Colds**)

FOOT PROBLEMS

I have received a multitude of letters on foot problems, so forgive me if they are not all included here, or this would become a book about feet! During an average lifetime, you will walk 71,000 miles. Feet contain 26 bones, 56 ligaments and 38 muscles, so there is plenty that can go wrong with our poor, often neglected feet.

FOOT PROBLEMS – FALLEN ARCHES

Try omniped supports invented by a foot specialist. They give all-round support to the feet. • **[LGF]**

FOOT PROBLEMS – HOT BURNING FEET

Poor circulation can cause this condition (*see* **Circulation**). People suffering from diabetes often have problems with the circulation or nerve supply to their feet. Improving circulation to the feet often relieves this problem.

Supplements
This problem can also be due to vitamin B deficiency especially B5 (pantothenic acid), so take a B complex daily with your main meal (*see* **General Health Hints**). Celluloid – sulphur compound – a good remedy when related to

itching and burning that is worse in bed. • [BLK]

Hints
Try using an Energy Roller, a wooden spiked roller developed over ten years by a reflexologist. It hurts a little initially, but stimulates pressure points. Many readers have reported increased circulation. For details, send an SAE to: Shakti Chakra, PO Box 3984, London SE12 0DZ. Acupuncture and reflexology are also very useful (*see* **Useful Information** *for further details*).

FOOT PROBLEMS – NUMB/TINGLING FEET
If you have numb and tingling feet, take the vitamins suggested under **Circulation**. Get plenty of exercise and try reflexology or acupuncture to help get your circulation moving (*see* **Useful Information** *for further details*).

FOOT PROBLEMS – SWOLLEN FEET AND ANKLES
A recurrent problem, usually in middle-aged women, which can cause great distress. A common cause of this problem is water retention caused by food sensitivity. Swollen ankles can also be caused by poor drainage of lymph fluid from the legs. Very occasionally, swollen feet and ankles may be the sign of more serious medical conditions such as heart, liver or kidney failure.

Diet
As a potassium-sodium imbalance can aggravate this problem, avoid all junk foods which contain a lot of salt and

promote swelling. Meat is high in sodium, especially red meat, so avoid all meat including chicken for six weeks. Include lots of potassium-rich foods in your diet, especially dark green vegetables like spinach, kale and cabbage, along with lots of fresh fruit, especially bananas. Eliminate salt completely from your cooking and do not add it to your food. Drink plenty of filtered water to help elimination and take regular exercise.

Supplements
Two celery seed extract, 1g of vitamin C as potassium ascorbate are good for drainage. Plus a good multi-vitamin daily. • [BC]

Try a silica and sulphur compound for three months to help improve the tone of your tissues, making them less likely to become waterlogged. On days when you are feeling particularly uncomfortable, take Herbal Fluid Balance containing dandelion leaves, which are a potassium-rich diuretic and help cleanse the liver. • [BLK]

Hints
Sit with your feet at hip level for 15 minutes every day, moving your feet back and forth to improve circulation. Rebounding (mini-trampolining) is especially good for boosting lymph drainage. Deep tissue lymphatic drainage can help if the problem is one of stagnant lymph. If the symptoms persist after following the advice given here for more than six weeks, ask your GP for a thorough check-up.

FROZEN SHOULDER
This condition is characterized by pain and limited move-ment in one, and very rarely both, shoulders. Frozen shoulder is due to inflammation in the muscles, ligaments

or tendons around the shoulder joint.

Diet
Avoid all acid-forming foods like meat, bread, cakes, biscuits and dairy products, which tend to increase inflammation in the body (*see* **General Health Hints**).

Supplements
Ligazyme, (containing calcium, vitamin C, bromelain, magnesium aspartate) to aid repair of the connective tissues. 2g of vitamin C daily along with mega GLA (an essential fatty acid), both of which are anti-inflammatory. Many people have reported benefits after taking alkymer shark liver oil capsules. • **[NC]**

Bromelain, turmeric and ginger are known as effective anti-inflammatory agents. • **[FSC]**

Hints
Traditionally, frozen shoulder is treated with physio-therapy. Alternatives are chiropractic and osteopathy, which are available on the National Health in some areas.

Try a magnetic plaster applied directly to the painful area, they have proved very successful in helping to alleviate pulled muscles and aching joints etc. For further information, contact MagnePlast on 0181 421 6525.

Algesic Cream, made from Indian herbs, relieves pain and inflammation. • **[HN]**

Make an ice pack by wrapping a small bag of frozen peas in a tea towel. Apply to the painful area for five minutes several times daily. Use your local swimming pool, as gentle movement in warm water loosens the shoulder.

Acupuncture and aromatherapy massage may also help alleviate some of the symptoms (*see* **Useful Information** *for further details*).

GALL-BLADDER PROBLEMS

The gall-bladder is a small sac about the size of a walnut that sits underneath and is connected to the liver. The gall-bladder's main function is to store bile which is made in the liver. The gall-bladder passes bile into the small bowel, where it helps break down fat during digestion. If the liver is overloaded with toxins, these tend to get dumped in the gall-bladder, a major cause of gall-bladder disease. The gall-bladder can be affected by gall-stones (*see page 127*), inflammation and infection. Each of these problems may produce pain on the right side and occasionally the centre of the abdomen.

Diet

Pain in the gall-bladder can sometimes be caused by food intolerance and it is wise to consult a nutritionist if you suffer from persistent gall-bladder related pain. In order to allow the gall-bladder to heal, it is necessary to let it rest. Avoid saturated fat in your diet by limiting red meat, dairy products, fried and processed foods. Stick to a good clean diet, made up of wholegrains, fruits and vegetables, and drink plenty of filtered water. Include one tablespoon of extra virgin olive oil, walnut oil or flax oil in your diet every day in salad dressings or add to vegetable juices. Lecithin granules extracted from soya beans emulsify fats – take one tablespoon daily over an oat-based cereal with low-fat rice milk (*see* **General Health Hints**).

Supplements

Both dandelion root and milk thistle extract help to eliminate gallstones and relieve gall-bladder problems in general, due to their ability to enhance bile production, flow and activity. Both herbs are easily available in capsule form.

Lipotropic Factors contains choline and inositol (both

part of the B group) and the amino acid methionine, all of which reduce the accumulation of fat in the liver, thereby reducing the tendency toward gall-bladder dysfunction. • **[S]**

GALL-BLADDER PROBLEMS – GALL-STONES

The gall-bladder gets rid of unwanted substances such as cholesterol and bilirubin into the bile duct, which in turn drains into the intestine. Gall-stones usually consist of a sediment made up of cholesterol, bilirubin and bile salts, and occur in individuals with excess cholesterol in the blood or as a result of stagnation in the gall-bladder.

Gall-stones often produce no symptoms at all, but can produce very intense bouts of abdominal pain. Other common symptoms include bloating, wind, nausea, and discomfort after rich, fatty food. Gall-stones affect 10% of the population over the age of 40 and are at least twice as common in women. People who are overweight have an increased risk of gall-stones. Recent research has shown that many gall-bladder patients suffer food allergies and once the allergen is found then surgery is often unnecessary (*see* **Allergies**).

Diet

Reduce all saturated fat intake like red meat and dairy products made from cows' milk. Try soya or rice milk instead which is non-dairy, low fat, sugar free and delicious. Cut down on the amount of alcohol, tea and coffee you drink. Avoid junk foods like hamburgers, which contain too much fat, salt and sugar, along with refined carbohydrates such as bread and cakes made with white flour. Avoid fatty, fried foods and eggs, which are known to trigger gall-bladder problems. Drink at least eight glasses of filtered water daily and increase your intake of extra virgin olive oil, which is thought to help dissolve the stones. Add plenty of fibre to your diet, which is found in fruit, vegetables, oat bran and wholegrain cereals like porridge, which can help to reduce the amount of fat absorbed from the diet.

Supplements
Herbs like milk thistle are useful for stimulating bile secretion and dissolving cholesterol. Lecithin granules increase the solubility of cholesterol and help reduce the formation of gall-stones. Use one tablespoon of lecithin daily on your cereal. People who suffer from gall-stones tend to be deficient in vitamin C and E, so take at least 1g of vitamin C and 200iu of vitamin E every day. • **[LGF]**

Reading
Natural Liver Therapy by Christopher Hobbs, £4.95, Botanica Press. Available from 0171 436 5122.

Hints
A reader sent the following gall-bladder flush remedy to me after being advised by a top American nutritionist. **Only attempt this remedy after discussing it with your GP.**

1. For five days prior to 'flush', drink 3½ pints (2 litres) of fresh, organic apple juice daily. Eat normally but avoid all saturated fats.
2. On the sixth day :
   Have no evening meal. At 9pm take one or two tablespoons of Epsom salts (a laxative) dissolved in 1–2 tablespoons of warm water.

   At 10pm mix 115g unrefined olive oil with 50g lemon juice. **Immediately** upon finishing the olive oil and juice go to bed and lie on your right side with your right knee drawn up towards your chin. Remain in this position for 30 minutes before going to sleep. This encourages the olive oil to drain from your stomach, helping contents of the gall-bladder and/or liver to move into the small intestine.

3. Next morning the stones should pass. They should be green in colour and soft like putty.

Potter's make GB tablets containing Black Root, Wahoo Bark, Kava and Burdock Root. Available from all good health stores.

GENERAL HEALTH HINTS

- Take regular, sensible exercise. Stick mainly to exercises such as brisk walking, cycling, light jogging, swimming, aerobics and aqua aerobics as these exercises have the most health-related benefits. You will be amazed at the difference regular exercise can make to your overall well-being. If you do nothing else, try to walk for 30 minutes daily.

- Make time for breakfast. Oat-based cereals or sugar-free muesli make an ideal breakfast for most people with oat, rice, soya, sheeps' or goats' milk.

- Drink at least six glasses of filtered or distilled water daily. Try not to drink too much fluid with food because it dilutes the digestive juices and pushes food too quickly through the system, which can lead to poor digestion of food and reduced absorption of nutrients.

- Cut down on tea, coffee, alcohol and caffeinated soft drinks which dehydrate the body. The additives and sugar in soft drinks can cause hyperactivity and different mood swings. Try herbal teas and dandelion coffee or barley drinks.

- Aim to eat three pieces of fresh organic fruit and three portions of vegetables or salad daily. The darker green the leaves, the more nourishing they are. Steam vegetables when possible, as boiling destroys vitamins. Many pesticides, especially the organophosphates (OPs) seep right through the vegetables and fruit and cannot be washed off. They are now linked with many cancers and lowered sperm counts. Therefore buy organic as much as possible. If we could all support organic farming then the price of organic produce will fall in time and there would be a huge reduction in the pesticides and chemicals in the air.

- Keep food simple – say no to rich foods with rich sauces and to fried foods (fried food is carcanogenic).
- Avoid pre-packaged, take-away and tinned foods whenever possible, as they are often full of salt, sugar and additives. Also a great majority of these foods are packed in aluminium containers, and aluminium has long been linked to Alzheimer's and senile dementia.
- Do not add salt to your food as it can aggravate water retention and cause blood pressure to rise. Our typical diet contains 9g of salt a day and it has been estimated that if we can reduce salt consumption to 3g per person per day it would save 70,000 deaths in Britain each year. Use a healthier alternative to salt like VitaSalt, which is available from BioCare.
- Do not become fanatical about fad diets. Everything in moderation and keep a balance of foods at all times for good nutrition. I love cakes but try and bake them only once a week! I bake cakes with butter which does not become rancid like some hard margarines when cooked. Use organic rice syrup, honey or fresh fruit instead of sugar. Or soak some dried fruits in warm water, drain, chop and add to the cake mix.
- Use extra virgin cold pressed olive oil in cooking and try walnut or cold pressed linseed oil for salad dressings. These oils have many health benefits from lowering cholesterol to aiding skin problems (*see* **Fats You Need to Eat**).
- Sit down to eat your meals; chew your food thoroughly to

aid digestion. Help digestion further by eating fruit between meals and not as a dessert. Fruit can ferment when eaten after a large meal causing wind and bloating.

- Cut down on any food containing refined sugar, which has little nutritional value and can cause hyperactivity, mood swings and depression. Avoid artificial sweeteners. If you are desperate for sugar use organic rice syrup, honey or molasses instead, which are found in any good health food store. As sugar depletes the body of chromium, take chromium to help reduce your sugar cravings.

- Cows' milk is often a problem for many people. Skimmed milk is higher in sugar (lactose) and many people are intolerant to this. Try oat, soya or rice milk which are non-dairy. Also use sheeps' or goats' products and eat plenty of live, low-fat yoghurt which contain beneficial gut bacteria and is rich in calcium.

- Use butter sparingly – although butter is better when baking cakes than margarine as it does not go rancid, when cooked. If using margarine, try to opt for a non-hydrogenated spread like Vitaquell or SuperSpread, available from good health stores and supermarkets.

- Wheat-based cereals, especially wheat bran, seem to cause bowel problems for many people. Use oat-based cereals, bran and bulgar instead. Pasta, which is made from a different type of wheat to other wheat-based products, seems to be better tolerated by most people.

- Try to avoid red meat which can putrefy in the gut and may contain antibiotic and chemical residues. Instead use free-range chicken or fresh fish.

- Avoid smoking and smoky atmospheres.

- Make time to relax. When we are stressed the body starts pumping the hormone adrenalin ready for the fight or flight response. Eventually this can cause us to blow a fuse. It can be a gastric fuse, leading to ulcers, or a heart fuse causing heart attacks, etc. The body and mind are one. If you are stressed, something has got to give in the end. Vitamins and diet alone will not keep you healthy. Stress is a major factor. Remember you are special, give yourself the odd treat and make space every day in your diary for yourself.

- Get plenty of fresh air and learn to breathe deeply; this aids relaxation. Deep breathing also helps to alkalize the body. Stress makes it too acid. Avoid over-exposure to the sun and wear a sunscreen in summer.

GENERAL SUPPLEMENTS FOR BETTER HEALTH

Supplements that I take daily as part of my health regime:

1. Chlorella, spirulina or blue-green algae. Because most of us eat too many acid-forming foods such as bread, cakes and protein, these super-rich green foods are packed with nutrients and provide an essential alkaline-forming balance as well as helping to detoxify the system. They are packed with concentrated nutrients usually found in fresh vegetables in a very digestible form. They are also a rich source of protein, iron, calcium, vitamin C, natural carotenes and fibre. I take a green supplement every day and believe this is the food of the future. Ask for details at your local health food store.

2. Many people do not understand that the body replenishes itself with food and they think that low-fat or no-fat diets are healthy. In fact we all need essential fats to function. Take one tablespoon of organic sunflower, pumpkin or sesame seeds every day or take an essential fatty acid supplement like evening primrose oil, starflower oil, GLA or linseed oil capsules. I take mine in the form of a cold pressed oil mixture which I mix into vegetable juice every day (*for details see* **Fats You Need to**

Eat). These oils protect your heart, digestive system, help your skin and improve brain function.

3. Most important of all, give yourself some worthwhile pollution protection and give your immune system a boost by taking 2g of vitamin C along with a good multi-vitamin/mineral each day. Additional essential anti-oxidant nutrients include natural vitamin E 100–400iu, plus 10–30mg of natural beta-carotene and 100–200mcg of selenium per day. These levels are not available in a normal diet. Prevention is always better than cure!

4. Take one acidophilus capsule daily. This helps to replenish the good bacteria in the gut and helps prevent many problems like candida, yeast infections, constipation and an over-acid system, caused not only by our foods but all the chemicals we inhale from the air.

GLANDULAR FEVER

Glandular fever is caused by the Epstein Barr virus and usually affects teenagers and young adults. Symptoms include severe sore throat, fever, swollen glands in the neck and feelings of malaise. The general malaise can persist for several months, as can the fatigue that also often accompanies the infection. Sometimes patients with glandular fever also develop a mild hepatitis caused by the Epstein Barr virus. Antibiotics are of no use because they are ineffective against viruses. Rest and good nutrition are vital to recovery, so take things easy to prevent a relapse.

Diet

Eat plenty of fresh vegetables like carrots, cabbage, broccoli, spinach and kale which are high in natural beta-carotene and magnesium. Incorporate an adequate intake of free-range poultry, fish, wholewheat bread, brown rice and oatmeal in your diet, but avoid sugar and sweetened foods and drinks, especially if you experience bloating (which may be an overgrowth of *Candida Albicans*, which often occurs with this condition). Sugar and refined carbohydrates can also suppress the function of the immune system, reducing its ability to fight the virus effectively. Drink at least six glasses of filtered water daily. Avoid alcohol and smoking.

Supplements
Magnesium levels often fall when we are ill, therefore take a calcium, magnesium and zinc complex daily along with 2g of vitamin C, which will all boost the immune system. Garlic is excellent for fighting infection. Take two capsules daily until symptoms ease. A multi-vitamin/mineral formula. Two acidophilus capsules daily to aid digestion and replace the good bacteria in the gut. • **[HN]**

Hints
A gradual return to normal life is necessary because over-activity too soon can cause a relapse. Check for possible iron deficiency with your doctor and take iron, if necessary (*see* **Anaemia**). If, after two months, your energy and appetite have not returned, contact a qualified nutritionist (*see* **Useful Information** *for further details*).

GOUT
Gout is a form of joint inflammation which is caused by high levels of uric acid in the blood causing crystal deposits in the joints. It is common in the big toe but can also affect other joints and the kidneys. Attacks may be precipitated by eating rich food, drinking too much alcohol on a regular basis, accident or trauma. Gout is basically a male disease; 95% of sufferers are men.

Diet
Avoid alcohol, anchovies, fatty fish, shellfish, red meat, oatmeal porridge, yeast, animal fats, lentils, cheese, coffee, tea, colas, and all sugary drinks and sweets which aggravate this condition. Stop adding salt to your meals and avoid tinned and pre-packed foods which often have a high salt content. Cherries are highly anti-inflammatory and, when they are in season, eat up to half a pound daily. Out of season, frozen or tinned cherries can be eaten. Eat copious amounts of fresh vegetables, fruits and their fresh juices, brown rice, millet, goats' milk and free-range eggs. Eating a ripe pear before each meal is an old French remedy. One reader found that when he gave up malted drinks, such as Horlicks, his gout disappeared. Drink at least eight glasses of filtered or bottled water daily to enable your kidneys to excrete as much uric acid as possible.

Supplements
Two celery seed extract capsules which increase the elimination of uric acid. 1g of vitamin C as magnesium ascorbate, magnesium, GLA, an essential fatty acid. Procydin complex containing pulp from cherries, blue-berries and blackberries, which are known to be powerful anti-oxidants. • [BC]

The herb Devil's Claw helps to neutralize the poisons causing the inflammation. Take daily whilst the attack lasts. **This should not be used during pregnancy. • [S]**

Reading
Curing Arthritis The Drug Free Way by Margaret Hills, £4.99, Sheldon Press.
The Natural Way with Arthritis and Rheumatism by Pat Young, £3.99, Element Books.

Hints
Do not take aspirin if taking anti-gout drugs.

GUMS (*see* **Bleeding Gums**)

HAEMORRHOIDS (*see* Piles)

HAIR LOSS

The health of the hair depends on the circulation to the root of the hair and the amount of nutrients present in the blood. Hair is composed of protein and minerals, and requires a healthy balanced diet for proper nourishment. It is thought that men lose hair on the top of their heads rather than the back and sides because the blood supply to the top of the scalp is reduced in comparison to lower down. When a person is very stressed, the scalp becomes very tight, resulting in restricted circulation which leads to the hair follicle becoming undernourished and the hair falling out.

Another important factor in hair loss is the male hormone testosterone. Although this is the hormone responsible for making men hairy during puberty, it also has a big part to play in hair loss from the scalp later in life. Hereditary factors are also important in hair loss. The more hair loss there is in your father, uncles and grandfathers, the more likely you are to lose your own hair. However, dietary supplements and regular, daily, firm scalp massage can help slow down hair loss.

Sudden hair loss in women can follow child birth and there are a number of other conditions like menopause and protein deficiency which can thin hair or cause it to fall out.

Diet

Stick to a well-balanced diet which includes plenty of fresh fruit, vegetables and proteins like beans and pulses. Drink plenty of water, at least six large glasses, daily. Low levels of zinc, iron and vitamin C are linked to hair loss. Natural sources of iron are egg yolks, green leafy vegetables, wholegrain breads and cereals and fish. Some people are unable to absorb all the nutrients from their food which can eventually cause hair loss (*see* **General Health Hints**).

Supplements

Vitamin E 300iu and zinc citrate for hair and nail growth. CT241, based upon natural extracts of marine food, especially for hair and nails, along with Colleginase (containing vitamin C, rutin, hesperidin, cellulase, silica and vitamins A and D) to strengthen connective tissue. Vitamin B, especially biotin and folic acid are helpful for hair growth. A digestive enzyme which helps absorption of nutrients. • [BC]

The herb Shen Min has been used in the Far East for thousands of years to help hair growth and many people have found this herb has helped reduce greying hair. For a brochure, call 0171 435 5911.

Reading

Coping with Sudden Hair Loss by Elizabeth Steele, £6.99, Thorsons.
Natural Solutions to Hair Loss and Scalp Problems by David Satchell, £5.50 (inc p&p), Allborough Press. To order from Action Against Alopecia, Tel/Fax: 01323 412723.

Hints

Take regular aerobic exercise which will stimulate your heart and circulation increasing oxygen flow, reducing stress and promoting scalp and hair health. Jojoba oil rubbed into the scalp can be very helpful for removing old layers of cells and impurities which can impede growth. Massage the scalp firmly for ten minutes each day to improve circulation; this really does help. Some readers suffering alopecia as a side-effect of severe stress found hypnotherapy really helped (*see* **Useful Information** *for details*).

Action Against Alopecia (membership £20 per annum) PO Box 2505, 3 Upperton Road, Eastbourne, East Sussex BN21 1AA. Tel: 01323 412723.

The Institute of Trichologists, 108 St Johns Hill, Clapham Junction, London SW11 1SW or call 0171 924 2195.

Natural Hair Products Ltd specialize in reversing hair loss in both men and women using a holistic approach which includes supplements. For details, call Mr Chris Pick who is a clinical nutritionist on 01798 343568.

✳ ❊ ✳

HALITOSIS (Bad Breath)

A common cause of bad breath is poor dental hygiene. See a qualified dental hygienist every six months. Use floss and mouthwash daily. Change your toothbrush regularly and clean your teeth at least twice a day. Poor digestion and the sluggish elimination of waste from the bowel are important causes of bad breath. Naturopaths believe that by improving digestion and bowel function, it is possible to eliminate bad breath.

Diet

Keep your diet as clean as possible by avoiding junk and sugar-based foods. Also avoid red meat, full fat milk, coffee and alcohol for a month to see if this helps. Food combining is a healthy way to eat and helps improve digestion. Smoking causes bad breath. The spice coriander is helpful for killing the bacteria, so use plenty in your cooking (*see*

General Health Hints).

Supplements
Two acidophilus bifidus capsules, plus a digestive aid containing a mixture of herbs and vegetable enzymes to be taken with each meal to aid digestion and absorption of nutrients. • **[BLK]**

Liquid chlorophyll is an excellent deodorizer for the intestinal tract. Take 5–6 drops daily. • **[NC]**

Reading
How To Improve Your Digestion and Absorption, by Christopher Scarfe, £2.50, ION Press.
New Self Help: Bad Breath by Leon Chaitow, £3.99, Thorsons.

Hints
Use a natural antiseptic mouthwash like tea tree oil. Add a few drops to warm water and use as a mouthwash, but do not swallow. With your doctor's permission, have a colonic irrigation which gently washes out the bowel helping to reduce toxicity (*see* **Useful Information** *for further details*).

A colon cleansing programme is available for home use by Natural Flow. For details, call 0181 874 1130.

Contact the Fresh Breath Centre, Conan Doyle House, 2 Devonshire Place, London W1N 1PA or call 0171 935 1666.

HANGOVERS (*see* Alcohol)

HAY FEVER (*see also* Allergies *and* Allergic Rhinitis)
Hay fever is caused by an allergic reaction to pollen and

usually causes red, itchy, watery eyes, sneezing and a runny or congested nose. Hay fever is sometimes confused with a condition called perennial rhinitis where symptoms are similar to hay fever but occur all year round. Common causes of perennial rhinitis include dust, pollution and food allergies.

Diet
To cleanse the system, keep the diet simple and avoid wheat, sugar, salt, food additives, coffee and mucus-forming foods like dairy produce made from cows' milk, which helps ease the strain on the upper respiratory system. Eat plenty of organic fruit and vegetables high in anti-oxidants, to boost the immune system. Try rice milk, which is non-dairy and low in fat. If symptoms are very severe, try an organic juice fast for one day each week to ease the load on the liver.

Supplements
To help prevent the onset of symptoms, begin this regime one month before symptoms usually start. 3g of vitamin C daily which has a natural antihistamine effect. The bioflavonoid quercetin helps to strengthen capillaries, thus preventing leakage into the bloodstream of the antibodies which cause the allergic reaction. • [LGF]

500mg of pantothenic acid (B5) with a B complex helps to relieve symptoms. Take 200iu of natural vitamin E which is anti-inflammatory, along with plenty of garlic, which helps to cleanse the sinuses. Bee pollen taken for several weeks prior to the start of the pollen season helps to reduce the allergic reaction.

Reading
Allergies by Stephen Terrass, £4.99, Thorsons.

Hints
Envirocare filters are designed to keep the air free of allergens. Expensive at £229 – but effective. For details, call 01344 874573.

Homeopathy has been successful in treating hay fever with remedies like *allium cepa* and *arundo*. Ask for details at your local homeopathic pharmacy or to find a qualified practitioner in your area (*see* **Useful Information** *for further details*). It is always a good idea to check for food allergies when you suffer severe hay fever and many foods 'cross-react' with pollen. See a kinesiologist who can help you to find specific allergens (*see* **Useful Information** *for details*).

HEALING AND HEALERS
Over the years I have heard an awful lot of people express negative opinions on this subject. Many people even accuse healers of using occult practices – to be frank, this is ludicrous. Consider the number of animals which respond to healing, even though they are not linked to any religion or belief and yet the healing works.

We all have energy fields around our bodies, most commonly known as auras. These can be photographed using Kirlian photography, which show many colours indicating the state of our internal health. If we are sick, then the aura is automatically affected. Healers aim to literally place healthy energy inside you and your aura, to re-balance your system and aid healing. Some people are born with a natural aptitude for maths or playing the piano, and are called geniuses or prodigies. Healers like Seka Nikolic and Matthew Manning, who have both been tested by scientists to measure their energy levels, were born with this energy and have gone on to fine tune and develop their ability throughout their lives.

People like me who love to give healing, but were not born with a natural aptitude can go for lessons and learn. Anyone can learn to heal people if they have a genuine desire to help and keep an open mind.

Spiritual healing is given by people who believe that the source of the healing energy comes from a divine origin, and they simply become a channel for this energy. (In much the same way that electrical sub-stations transfer electricity from the generating source to the consumer.) People seeking healing should always contact a reputable organization such as The National Federation of Spiritual Healers (NFSH) who will put you in touch with an accredited registered healer who has received thorough training.

Reading

Dr Dan Benor is a practising psychotherapist and healer who has published more than 150 scientific studies of healing in humans and animals. *Healing Research* by Dr Daniel Benor, Helix Books. Volume One is £29.60; Volume Two is £22.00. To order, call 01524 68765. Highly recommended for any doctor who would like to know more about healing and healers.

The Complete Healer by David Furlong, £9.99, Piatkus Books.

Light Emerging, The Journey Of Personal Healing by an ex-NASA space scientist who is now a healer, Barbara Ann Brennan, £16.99, Bantam. To order call 0171 436 5122. Her books on healing are well worth reading.

Spiritual Healing: Everything You Want To Know, by Liz Hodgson, £7.99, Piatkus Books.

Your Hands Can Heal by Ric A Weinman, £4.99, Thorsons.

Hints

For information, contact The NFSH, Old Manor Farm Studio, Church Street, Sunbury-on-Thames, Middlesex TW16 6RG. To obtain the referral line for your nearest two

142

healers call 0891 616080. For general information, call 01932 783164. There are some excellent healers affiliated to The Hale Clinic in London. For details, call 0171 631 0156.

HEARTBURN (*see* **Acid Stomach, Indigestion** *and* **Low Stomach Acid**)

HEART DISEASE (*see also* **Angina, Circulation, Cholesterol** *and* **High Blood Pressure**)

Heart disease is the number one killer in the Western world. A lot of people think that heart disease is a predominantly male condition. In fact, heart disease is the most common cause of death in women too! The heart, like any muscle, needs its own blood supply and gets this via three main vessels called the coronary arteries which can be seen on the surface of the heart. Gradually over time, one or more of these arteries can become blocked with a fatty substance. If an artery blocks off completely, some of the heart muscle may die during a heart attack. Typical symptoms of a heart attack include a severe pressing band of pain across the chest which can spread up the neck into the jaw, or across the shoulders and down into the left arm. The pain can be associated with sweating, breathlessness and a feeling of nausea. **Immediate medical aid should be sought.**

A hundred years ago, heart attacks were rare, but today many people lead sedentary lives and eat diets high in fat and sugar and low in essential nutrients. Recent tests at Cambridge University testing 2,000 heart attack patients found that if a person takes between 400–800iu of vitamin E every day they are 75% less likely to suffer another heart

143

attack. In an average daily diet, eating more than 50iu would be rare, therefore it would be wise to take at least 400iu of natural source vitamin E every day.

Diet
Wholefood diet rich in vegetables, fruits, grains and fresh nuts (especially walnuts) and seeds. Avoid red meat and dairy products made from cows' milk that are high in saturated fat and salt and can raise blood pressure. Especially avoid all transfats found in hydrogenated vegetable oils and hard margarines. Use a healthier spread like Vitaquell. Never use refined oils, which are like white sugar – all the goodness has been removed in the processing. Avoid any pre-packaged foods which contain hydrogenated ingredients. Include oily fish at least twice a week in your diet or take fish oil supplements. Eat plenty of fresh garlic as it thins the blood and aids circulation. Make salad dressings from organic walnut oil, olive oil or linseed (flax) oil (*see* **General Health Hints**).

Supplements
1g of vitamin C and 500mg of the amino acid lysine can help to reverse blockages in the arteries. 400iu of vitamin E. Lack of magnesium is associated with an increased risk for heart attacks and strokes, therefore take a calcium, magnesium and zinc complex daily. B Complex plus an anti-oxidant formula and 30–60mg of Co-enzyme Q10 are all beneficial to the heart. Essential fats are also vital for a healthy heart (*see* **Fats You Need to Eat**).

Reading
Beat Heart Disease Without Surgery by Jillie Collings, £6.99, Thorsons.
Heart Health For Women by Felicity Smart & Dr Diana Holdright, £6.99, Thorsons.
Super Nutrition For A Healthy Heart by Patrick Holford,

£2.50. To order, call 0181 877 9993.

Hints
For a healthy heart, don't become overweight. Take regular exercise, which not only aids the heart, but reduces stress, which is a major cause of heart problems. Stress thickens the blood and is a major trigger for heart problems. Tai Chi and yoga are great forms of exercise for reducing stress. See a doctor who is also a nutritionist to re-balance your diet and help you to prevent heart disease (*see* **Useful Information** *for further details*).

   Contact the British Heart Foundation by sending an SAE to: 14 Fitzhardinge Street, London W1H 4DH or by calling 0171 935 0185.

HERPES
There are two types of *herpes simplex* virus: Type I herpes causes cold sores, (*see* **Cold Sores**); Type II is sexually transmitted and is the most common. It can range from a silent infection to serious inflammation of the liver causing extreme pain and swelling in the genital area accompanied by fever. You never get rid of the virus once you have it, but you can keep attacks under control by taking supplements and eating a healthier diet.

Diet
(*See dietary section under* **Cold Sores**.)

Supplements
Cat's claw tea is helpful for both types of herpes. Drink it daily to boost your energy and immunity. Take 1g of the amino acid lysine which helps inhibit the virus, along with 1g of vitamin C. Take at the onset of symptoms. Licrogel is

a special gel that cools and speeds the healing of herpes sores if they do develop. • [HN]

Hints
As genital herpes is sexually transmitted, use condoms and practise safe sex.

HIATUS HERNIA
The gullet or oesophagus takes food from the mouth to the stomach and passes through a sheet of muscle called the diaphragm. A hiatus hernia occurs when part of the stomach pushes up through the diaphragm and allows acid to escape into the gullet causing heartburn and indigestion, especially when lying down.

Diet
Avoid alcohol, coffee, tea, sugar, chocolate, artificial additives and artificial sweeteners. Try dandelion coffee and caffeine-free herb and fruit teas. Avoid heavy, rich meals and never rush food as stress can cause the digestive system to shut down. Steam, grill or boil but don't fry food as it is hard to digest. Chew thoroughly and avoid drinking with meals (*see* **Acid Stomach**). Eat a live, low-fat yoghurt daily to help soothe the lining of the digestive tract. Food combining is usually very beneficial for anyone who has a hiatus hernia (*see* **General Health Hints**).

Supplements
Lecithin granules emulsify fats and one tablespoon can be taken daily. 1g of vitamin C with bioflavonoids, plus calcium and magnesium to calm the digestive tract. 200iu of vitamin E and garlic which is very cleansing. A digestive enzyme taken with main meals will help to improve the

digestive process and avoid indigestion.

2g of the amino acid glutamine taken daily for two months helps to repair the gut and any ulceration. Aloe juice can be taken before each meal to help rebuild the digestive lining. • [HN]

Reading
Food Combining In 30 Days by Kathryn Marsden, £4.99, Thorsons.
New Self Help: Hiatus Hernia by Joan Lay, £2.99, Thorsons.

Hints
A programme of relaxation would be of benefit as it reduces stress and aids digestion. Do not exercise immediately after eating. Try swimming, walking or yoga every day for at least 30 minutes.

HIGH BLOOD PRESSURE

High blood pressure increases your risk of heart disease and is *the* most important risk factor for stroke. It is generally accepted that a blood pressure of 140/90 or below is healthy. A blood pressure of 150/100 or more, is classified as raised. Anything in between is normally referred to as borderline raised. Being overweight and lack of exercise increases your risk of high blood pressure. Dietary factors are also important; there is now a clear and proven link between salt in the diet and blood pressure. Stop smoking as nicotine contracts blood vessels. Stress thickens the blood and can drive up blood pressure.

Diet
Researchers in the Netherlands have found that mineral salts containing magnesium and potassium can help to

reduce blood pressure. A drastic reduction of salt (sodium) was also found to be beneficial. In the West we eat far too much salt, especially in processed foods. Our typical diet contains 9g of salt a day and it has been estimated that if we can reduce salt consumption by 6g per person per day it would save 70,000 deaths in Britain each year. Use a healthier salt like VitaSalt, made by BioCare.

To keep your arteries as healthy as possible, eat a diet low in saturated fats and high in mono-unsaturated fats like extra virgin olive oil or linseed oil, which are ideal for salad dressings (*see* **Fats You Need to Eat**). Eat plenty of high fibre foods, like wholegrains, pulses, wholemeal bread and potatoes (not fried). For healthy fats, eat oily fish like mackerel, salmon, tuna and sardines at least twice a week. Studies involving a higher potassium intake show that potassium from the diet helps to lower blood pressure. Include more bananas, cantaloupe melons, tomatoes, green leafy vegetables and potatoes in your diet as they are high in potassium. Cut down on any drinks containing caffeine and alcohol. High levels of lead which can contaminate drinking water are known to contribute to hypertension. If you live in an area with soft water, buy a good water filter (*see* **General Health Hints**).

Supplements

Garlic with your main meal. Bio-magnesium, as low levels of magnesium are often found in high blood pressure sufferers. 1g of vitamin C daily. Vitamin E 400iu daily to protect the heart. Co-enzyme Q10 is an important enzyme found in organ meats which is often lacking in later life and 30–50mg taken regularly helps to reduce high blood pressure. GLA is an essential fatty acid for keeping blood healthy (*see* **Fats You Need to Eat**).

CH192 contains chromium, digestive enzymes and niacin (B3) which helps to bind cholesterol nutrients to strengthen the heart muscles and aid circulation. • [BC]

Reading
Recipes For High Blood Pressure by Maggie Pannell, £5.99, Thorsons.
High Blood Pressure by Dr Caroline Shreeve, £4.99, Thorsons.
Super Nutrition For A Healthy Heart by Patrick Holford, £2.50. To order, call 0181 877 9993.

Hints
Cayenne pepper is anti-hypertensive. Use one teaspoon daily in cooking. Hot, but helpful! **(Do not use if you suffer from stomach ulcers.)** Stress, anxiety and excess weight can play a major role in raising blood pressure. Try yoga, Tai Chi and deep breathing, which all help to lower blood pressure. Exercise is vital in controlling this condition. With your doctor's permission start walking briskly for 30 minutes daily. Try Ruthmol instead of table salt, which is potassium- and not sodium-based. Rosemary and nettle tea sipped regularly can help to lower blood pressure.

HIRSUTISM (*see also* **Body Hair, Excessive**)

HYPERACTIVITY

Hyperactivity is a condition which occurs predominantly in children, although the symptoms can occasionally extend into adulthood. Children who suffer from hyperactivity are typically unable to concentrate or sit still, suffer severe mood swings and are difficult to quieten down. Sleep is a major problem for hyperactive children. Hyperactivity is almost always associated with too much sugar and artificial food additives in the diet. Many children's drinks and even toothpastes are packed with artificial colourings and additives. Excessive exposure to neurotoxins such as lead, along with deficiencies in nutrients like chromium, zinc and essential fats can have a quite dramatic effect on their behavioural patterns.

Diet
Diet should be low in sugar, salt and refined foods like cakes, biscuits, white bread, chocolate and cola type drinks. Concentrate more on wholefoods including organic vegetables, fruits, wholegrain cereals, fish and free range chicken. Food sensitivity is another common factor in hyperactive children. The most common offenders seem to be wheat, dairy products, eggs and citrus fruits (*see* **Allergies** *and* **General Health Hints.**)

Supplements
Omega 3 and omega 6 are essential fats needed for hyperactive kids. Essential Balance oil for children, which contains a perfect balance of the omega 3 and 6 oils with a natural butterscotch flavouring, can be added to shakes and desserts. Dinochews multi/mineral has the correct level of zinc and other minerals needed to help hyperactive youngsters. • [HN]

Reading
The Allergy Survival Guide by Jane Houtton, £10.99, Vermilion.
How to Get A Peaceful Night's Sleep by Heather Welford, £4.99, Thorsons.
The Hyperactive Child by Belinda Barnes & Irene Colquhoun, £3.50.
Hyperactive Child Cookbook by Dulcie Roberts and Janet Ash, £6.50.
The above two books are available from HACSG, 71 Whyke Lane, Chichester, West Sussex PO19 2LD.

Hints

For further information, send an SAE to: The Hyperactive Children's Support Group, 71 Whyke Lane, Chichester, West Sussex PO19 2LD or call 01903 725182 between 10am and 1pm.

If you cannot afford an allergy blood test, take your child to see a kinesiologist, who uses muscle testing to detect food and environmental allergens (*see* **Useful Information** *for further details*).

INCONTINENCE (*see also* **Bladder** *and* **Prostate Problems**)

Urine can leak out when the bladder is put under pressure i.e. when you laugh, cough, sneeze or exert yourself. This type of problem is referred to as stress incontinence and is usually associated with weakness in a sheet of muscle called the pelvic floor. Exercise helps keep the pelvic floor strong and childbirth tends to weaken it. I have received hundreds of letters from embarrassed women and I have to confess that on this one ladies, I personally resorted to surgery. I had two weeks off work, found a good gynaecologist who specialized in this surgery and had myself stitched up. I have to say that doing the Jane Fonda aerobic workout is much easier these days!

Diet

Incontinence can be aggravated by cystitis-like symptoms which are often due to candida or food intolerance (*see* **Cystitis** *and* **Candida** *for more details and* **General Health Hints**).

Supplements

Take a multi-vitamin/mineral plus 1g of vitamin C. Calcium, magnesium citrate complex to aid muscle control. • [S]

Reading
Bladder Problems by Rosy Reynold, £3.99, Thorsons.
Understanding Incontinence by Dorothy Mandelstam, £6.95, Chapman & Hall.

Hints
Strengthening the pelvic floor can reduce or eliminate stress incontinence. The pelvic floor contracts when you tighten the muscles you would use to try and stop your urine flow. Hold this for three seconds and repeat a total of five times. This whole exercise can be repeated up to ten times a day. Gradually, you should notice that the exercise becomes easier and easier to do, and any problems with stress incontinence should improve.

Try using a set of vaginal cones, containing weights to help strengthen the muscles. For information on the Aquaflex System, call 0800 614086. There is also a helpline available on 0800 526177.

Contact the Continence Foundation, 2 Doughty Street, London WC1N 2PH. This charity provides information and advice and has a helpline on 0191 213 0050, Monday–Friday 9am–6pm.

An osteopath or chiropractor can check the alignment of bones in the pelvic area. When bones are out of balance it can affect urine flow for men and women. Acupuncture has proved helpful to some readers, as has aromatherapy (*see* **Useful Information** *for further details*). Incontinence in children is often linked to an allergic reaction (*see* **Allergies**). Many people report that when they stop using toothpaste and drinking water containing fluoride their urine problems stop after a few weeks.

INDIGESTION (*see also* Acid Stomach, Low Stomach Acid *and* Hiatus Hernia)

Indigestion is usually a sign that the digestive system is having difficulty coping with the food. This is often due to a lack of stomach acid and/or digestive enzymes in the small intestine. This can be made worse if you eat quickly and don't chew food thoroughly. Over-eating, drinking with meals, eating bad food combinations or eating when stressed, all exacerbate indigestion.

Diet

Avoid too much coffee, tea, alcohol, chocolate, sugar, red meat, citrus fruits, onions and peppers, which are all known to cause indigestion. Chew thoroughly, avoid drinking with meals and eat little and often, rather than having one or two big meals in a day. Food combining is an excellent way to help reduce the symptoms of indigestion by making life easy for the digestive system. Fruit should not be eaten with other foods, if possible. Fruit passes through the stomach quite quickly but other foods like proteins and starches take much longer. Fruit ferments when eaten on top of a large meal producing gas and causing indigestion. Always eat fruit on an empty stomach and wait at least half an hour before eating any other food.

Supplements

Chlorella is a supplement made from concentrated sea algae. In addition to being a good source of nutrients, it is particularly rich in plant-based enzymes which, when taken with food, can help towards proper digestion and assimilation. If flatulence is particularly troublesome or if indigestion is recurring, then take a digestive enzyme with every meal. • [NC].

Take two acidophilus capsules daily for six weeks which

helps replenish good bacteria in the gut, which in turn aids the digestive process.

Ginger capsules are very useful for indigestion, 500–1,000mg as needed.

Reading
How To Improve Your Digestion and Absorption, by Christopher Scarfe, £2.50, ION.

Hints
The homeopathic remedies *calc phos* and *phosphorus* can ease heartburn. See a homeopath or a nutritionist who will help re-balance your system (*see* **Useful Information** *for further details*).

INFERTILITY

Sperm counts have dropped 50% in the last 50 years. One in six couples in Britain experiences problems with fertility. In one third of these cases the problem is with the man, one third is with the woman and in the remaining third, the problem is with both partners. If the male sperm count is low, this can sometimes be due to an infection such as mumps. A low sperm count can be due to poor nutrient status and/or environmental poisons such as lead, mercury or cadmium. Excessive smoking and drinking also reduce sperm counts substantially. Many scientists now believe that sperm counts in the Western world are dropping because of the oestrogen-like compounds in the environment such as herbicides and pesticides.

In women, infertility can sometimes be due to blockages in the tubes which transmit eggs from the ovaries to the womb (fallopian tubes). This is usually due to an infection such as pelvic inflammatory disease. Sometimes there is a problem with ovulation, usually due to hormonal imbalance. Nutritional deficiencies, particularly in the minerals zinc and magnesium and/or environmental pollutants, are also common causes of infertility in women. A significant number of infertile women suffer from candida and clearing this can often result in a successful pregnancy (*see* **Candida**). Many women are under too much stress which causes the release of adrenalin. Their endocrine system eventually becomes exhausted which can prevent conception from taking place.

Diet

Keep the diet clean and devoid of any artificial additives, stimulants and sugar. Caffeine can adversely affect reproduction; avoid too much coffee and tea. Drink herbal teas and dandelion coffee. Alcohol should be kept to an absolute minimum and preferably stopped six months prior to conception. The diet should be based around organic wholegrains like brown rice and wholewheat pasta, fresh fruits and vegetables. Eat a little fresh oily fish and free-range chicken. Zinc is vital for both partners; therefore eat plenty of pumpkin and sesame seeds which are high in zinc. Eat plenty of soya products like tofu, fennel and alfalfa which contain oestrogen-like substances thought to be beneficial. Tap water is often contaminated by chemicals; invest in a good water filter system like Watersimple. Further details are available from The Fresh Water Filter Company, Carlton House, Aylmer Road, London E11 3AD or call 0181 558 7495.

Supplements

Omega 3 and omega 6 oils are beneficial for reproductive systems. To get the balance right, take one tablespoon of Essential Balance Oil daily. Made from organic linseeds, pumpkin and sunflower seeds which are also high in vitamin E and beta carotene. • **[HN]**

Orchi-Zinc is important for reproductive gland function. 97% of referred couples for pre-conceptual care show evidence of zinc deficiency. Zinc, magnesium and the amino acid arginine are needed for healthy sperm. • **[NC]**

Vitamin B complex is vital for hormone control and calcium and magnesium, plus 5,000iu of vitamin A daily are needed for egg and sperm production. • **[S]**

There is a pregnancy pack which includes all the vitamins and minerals needed by women who are trying to conceive, for pregnancy and through breast-feeding. Made by Health Plus. For details, call 01323 737374 .

Reading
Infertility by Roger Neuberg, £7.99, Thorsons.
Infertility by Maggie Jones, £6.99, Piatkus Books.
Optimum Nutrition by Patrick Holford, £5.95, ION Press. (Also from ION Press, read Volume 9, Number 2 of their magazine, reference *Fertility*.)
The Natural Way: Fertility by Belinda Whitworth, £3.99, Element Books.

Hints
Avoid contact with all pesticides and eat only organic foods. As both partners' vitamin and mineral status need to be carefully checked, always consult a nutritional doctor (*see* **Useful Information** *for details*). Contact Foresight, who specialize in giving couples information about how to plan for a healthy pregnancy and increase fertility naturally. The service includes nutritional status analysis, though this is usually done in consultation with a recognized Foresight practitioner. Foresight can be contacted by writing to: 28 The Paddock, Godalming, Surrey, GU7 1XD.

INSECT BITES

Apart from the obvious discomfort they can cause, insect bites can occasionally transmit serious diseases and cause severe allergic reactions like analphylactic shock. If you know that you, your partner or child has a particular allergy to stings and bites, be sure to ask your GP for a supply of anti-histamines. In extreme cases, it is sometimes essential for sufferers to have adrenalin injections on hand.

Diet
Eating fresh garlic has a natural repellent effect.

Supplements
Thiamine (vitamin B1) and zinc, which when excreted through the body give off an odour which repels insects; but to be effective, a dosage of 100mg of thiamine, three times daily would be necessary and at least 60mg of zinc. Thiamine is best taken as part of a B complex preparation to prevent imbalance in these vitamins. Many people report that by taking brewer's yeast complex they stay free from bites. The herb feverfew taken daily has worked well for many readers.

Hints
Try an essential oil preparation for repelling insects. Mix ten drops of lavender oil, ten drops of orange oil, five drops of eucalyptus, five drops of citronella and ten drops of neem oil (the neem tree in India is well known to repel mosquitoes) into a base of 50ml of apricot or almond oil. Use sparingly on exposed areas of skin, most especially ankles and wrists. You should be able to find these oils at any good health store or call 0171 436 5122. Alternatively, place a few drops of this combination onto any light bulbs in the room (before switching bulbs on), as the aroma will again act as a repellent. Avoid wearing any perfumed toiletries at night and use cotton night clothes that cover the arms and wrists.

Use lemon grass candles in the evening to act as a repellent.

INSOMNIA (*see also* **Sleeping Pills**)

Insomnia affects one in five people in the UK today. I have been a chronic insomniac for nearly 20 years and I know exactly how it feels to be wide awake at 3am, worrying about having to be up early. For me and many other sufferers, the problem is an inability to shut down and let go of all the thoughts that are going through our minds. The simple fact is that once you are able to let go of these thoughts, sleep is much more likely. If you sleep well when you go on holiday then you are most likely a highly-stressed person who thinks too much! A good way to overcome this problem is meditation, which enables you to relax and feel more peaceful (*see* **Meditation**), or try practising some form of relaxation technique. Sleeping pills may work in the short term, but over extended periods they begin to lose their effectiveness and actually make sleeping more difficult as they can alter the delicate chemistry in the brain. Also, there is always the risk of addiction with long-term use.

Diet

Avoid caffeine in the afternoon and evening as this is a common cause of insomnia. Don't eat late at night, as digestion takes up a lot of energy and can keep you awake. Carbohydrates like pasta, potatoes and brown rice make a better evening meal than protein because they are easier to digest and also have a more sedating effect on the brain. Alcohol, although it can help you get off to sleep, can also cause you to wake in the middle of the night and is best avoided.

Supplements

Melatonin is a hormone secreted by the pineal gland which regulates our internal body clock. Melatonin production is suppressed if we do not get enough natural daylight which can disrupt sleep patterns (*see* **SAD Syndrome**).

Melatonin has been widely used to help people overcome jet lag and to regulate the internal body clock. It is also an important anti-oxidant nutrient. In the UK melatonin is not licensed as an aid to sleep without a prescription. If your doctor is willing to prescribe melatonin (which is identical in molecular structure to the hormone produced in your brain), it can be filled through certain health stores. For details, call 0171 436 5122. Before going to bed, place one 3mg tablet under the tongue. Melatonin can be purchased over the counter in Ireland and America. For further information, plus a free fact sheet, call PharmWest in Ireland on 00 353 1862 1309.

Sleeping pills deplete the body of vitamin B, therefore take a B complex every day. Many people who cannot sleep are deficient in magnesium, calcium and zinc. • **[FSC]**

Bioforce make a tincture called Dormesan made from herbs such as lemon balm, hops and valerian, all of which have sedative properties. Excellent for people who tend to sleep easily initially and then wake during the small hours.

Kava kava root from a Polynesian plant is widely used as a herbal supplement to help people to feel calmer. It should be taken regularly at bedtime and has a cumulative effect after four to six weeks. • **[S]**

Reading

Restful Sleep by Deepak Chopra, £7.99, Rider.
Melatonin: Your Body's Natural Wonder Drug, by Russell J Reiter and Jo Robinson, £19.50, Bantam.
Stress, Anxiety and Insomnia by Michael Murray, £9.95, Prima Press.
A Good Night's Sleep. Free – send two first class stamps to

Green Library, 9 Rickett Street, London SW6 1RU or call them on 0171 385 0012.

Hints
Don't read any work papers close to bed-time; it stimulates your mind. Read an easy novel to take your mind off work and the stresses of the day. If you can't sleep, don't panic. Get up and do something relaxing like reading a few more pages until you start to relax and let go; then go back to bed. Don't try to go to sleep, let yourself fall asleep naturally. Turn the bedside clock to the wall, then you will not panic about the time. Put some lavender oil on a tissue and inhale before bed. Drink camomile tea at night. Try Australian Bush Flower Essences (Insomnia Blend) containing crowea, boronia and black-eyed Susan. A few drops on the tongue before bed aid sleep by slowing an over-active mind. For further details, contact Serena Smith on 0171 431 6153.

Many readers have found Isocones, which work on pressure points, helpful in aiding natural sleep. Made by Sea Bands. For details, call the Nutri Centre on 0171 436 5122. Reflexology, homeopathy, acupuncture and hypnotherapy have all proved useful in restoring natural sleep patterns. *Chamomilla*, the homeopathic remedy is good for insomnia that occurs after a mental upset (*see* **Useful Information** *for further details*).

Persistent insomnia can also be caused by food allergies in which case it would be wise to consult a doctor who is also a qualified nutritionist (*see* **Useful Information** *for further details*).

INTERMITTENT CLAUDICATION (*see also* **Angina** *and* **Heart Disease**)
This condition is characterized by pain in the legs, usually in

the calves on walking. It is caused by blockages in the arteries supplying blood to the legs. Intermittent claudication is essentially angina of the legs.

Diet
(*See under* **Angina** *and* **General Health Hints**.)

Supplements
1g of vitamin C, plus 500mg of the amino acid lysine, both three times daily to help reverse the hardening of the arteries. 300iu of natural vitamin E to help reduce stickiness in the blood and aid circulation. Magnesium 400mg daily to help keep the arteries open. Essential fatty acids are vital for this condition (*see* **Fats You Need to Eat**).

Reading
(*See under* **Angina**.)

Hints
Although exercise may be initially painful, with your doctor's permission, start walking for a few minutes each day, gradually increasing to 30 minutes or more. This helps to increase circulation in the legs.

IRRITABLE BOWEL SYNDROME – IBS (*see also* **Diverticular Disease**)

Also known as spastic colon, IBS is a disorder characterized by abdominal and digestive symptoms which often cannot be explained by the conventional medical establishment. Typical symptoms include bloating, wind, abdominal discomfort, and constipation and/or diarrhoea which are all exacerbated by stress. IBS is very often due to an imbalance in the organisms that live in the gut and this often includes an overgrowth in yeast (*see* **Candida**). It can also be due to food sensitivity. Occasionally, symptoms may be due to a potentially serious condition such as Crohn's disease or ulcerative colitis, therefore always consult your doctor before attempting to self-treat.

Diet

If you suspect food sensitivity, then remove the suspect(s) from your diet to see what effect this has. Likely culprits are wheat and dairy products made from cows' milk. Base your diet around brown rice, potatoes, poultry, fish, organic fresh fruit and vegetables. If symptoms are severe, also avoid grains such as oats and rye. If you suspect yeast is a problem then try going on a anti-yeast diet (*see* **Candida**) for a month, as this is very likely to help the symptoms. Fructose and sorbitol are sweeteners which affect some sufferers quite badly, so check food labels carefully.

Supplements

Absorption is very often a problem for IBS sufferers, therefore you may not be getting enough nutrition from the food you eat, so take liquid multi-vitamins which are easily absorbed each day.

If candida is present then Candicidin **(not to be taken if pregnant)** and the healthy bacteria bio-acidophilus are often effective. Take a digestive enzyme with main meals which will help to ease symptoms. NT188 containing B vitamins and herbs like passiflora to calm the nerves. • **[BC]**

The amino acid glutamine, aloe vera juice and essential fats found in linseed oil (*see* **Fats You Need to Eat**), all help to heal the lining of the digestive system. • **[HN]**

Reading

Irritable Bowel and Diverticulosis by Shirley Trickett, £5.99, Thorsons.
Irritable Bowel Syndrome Special Diet Cookbook by Jill Davies

and Ann Page-Wood, £5.99, Thorsons.
Aloe Vera – The Legendary Healer by Alasdair Barcroft, £6.99,
Souvenir Press. Available from 0181 871 5083.

Hints
Gentle exercise like yoga, swimming or walking every day
helps with IBS as exercise lowers stress levels, which can
exacerbate the problem. A daily banana has helped many
IBS sufferers.

Call the Woman's Nutritional Advisory Service, who
offer help to IBS sufferers, on 01273 487366.

KIDNEY STONES
Kidney stones are usually made of insoluble crystals of
minerals which are found in the urine. Most stones are
formed from calcium salts, but stones made of other
substances, such as uric acid, are also known. Stones form in
the kidney, the bladder or in the tubes which connect the
kidneys to the bladder known as the urethra, and they can
cause excruciating pain. Stones make infection more likely
and their formation can sometimes be triggered by
infection. If you suffer persistent lower back pain near the
waist line or pass blood in your urine, see your GP.

Diet
Because most stones are high in calcium and oxalic acid,
avoid any foods which are rich in these substances;
beetroot, cocoa, chocolate, currants, dried figs, rhubarb,
parsley, spinach, tea, blackberries, gooseberries, oranges,
strawberries, raspberries, carrots, green beans, onions,
cucumber and lemon peel. Keep dairy products, especially
full cream cows' milk, to a minimum. Use non-dairy rice
milk. Eat less animal protein, salt and sugar, as these

increase calcium levels in the blood. Take two tablespoons of virgin olive oil daily in cooking or salad dressings. Drink at least six glasses of filtered water daily and avoid alcohol (*see* **General Health Hints**).

Supplements

Magnesium helps to prevent calcium depositing in the kidneys and joints, so take a daily supplement of 400mg of magnesium, along with a B complex and 25mg of B6 which helps to normalize oxalic metabolism. Take a multivitamin and mineral. • [Q]

Lecithin helps to dissolve kidney stones as it emulsifies bad fats. Take one tablespoon daily over cereal.

Reading

The Principles Of Nutritional Therapy by Linda Lazarides, £5.99, Thorsons.

Hints

Inactivity tends to keep calcium in the kidneys, therefore regular exercise such as swimming, walking or cycling will aid prevention of more stones forming.

LEG ULCERS (*see also* **Circulation**)

A common problem among the over-60s caused by restricted circulation, and lack of oxygen and nutrients to the skin. Ulcers are more common in diabetics due to changes in circulation and the nervous supply to the skin.

Diet

Increase the amount of dark green leafy vegetables in your diet such as cabbage, kale and broccoli which contain high levels of beta-carotene and essential vitamins. Eat plenty of natural low-fat, live yoghurt and try to eat free-range poultry instead of red meat; also add fish, wholemeal bread, brown rice and oatmeal to your diet. Include plenty of fresh garlic as it is anti-bacterial and aids healing (*see* **General Health Hints**).

Supplements

A multi-vitamin and mineral. Zinc citrate, as zinc is vital for skin healing, take daily for two months. Flax oil is excellent for skin, take one tablespoon daily stirred into fresh vegetable or fruit juice. 2g of vitamin C and natural beta-carotene complex. The amino acid glutamine helps rapid healing of ulcers. • **[HN]**

Hints

Nutraderm, a skin treatment rich in vitamins C and A, should help heal ulcers. Apply it to the skin around the ulcer and apply it a little closer to the ulcer each day. • **[HN]**

Try Bach Rescue Remedy cream once the skin starts to heal – from good health stores.

Raise legs above hip level when resting and move feet backwards and forwards slowly to increase circulation in lower legs. Try and walk for at least 15 minutes daily.

Many readers have found that acupuncture and reflexology improve circulation.

Magnet therapy is known to increase circulation. For details of magnetic products, send an SAE to: Acar-Sud, Westfield House, Hampton Court Road, East Molesey, Surrey KT8 9BX or call 0181 977 1699.

LICHEN PLANUS

A chronic condition of the skin and mucous membranes, such as the lining of the mouth, thought to be caused by a virus. It has features in common with other skin problems like eczema and psoriasis. The sores on the skin are often localized on the wrists and ankles, but it can be widespread.

Diet
Keep to a healthy diet and avoid all dairy products made from cows' milk; instead use soya or rice products and vegetable margarines like Vitaquell or SuperSpread. Avoid stimulants such as vinegar, alcohol and hot spicy foods. Also reduce or avoid apples, cherries, pineapples, mushrooms, coffee, honey, red meat, chocolate, ice-cream, sugar and sugary foods. Eat oily fish like salmon or mackerel at least twice a week, along with plenty of vegetables, raw whenever possible (*see* **General Health Hints**).

Supplements
Vitamin B12 plus NutriGuard Forte containing beta-carotene, selenium and vitamins A, C and E to protect and restore skin and tissues against infection. Mega GLA is an essential fatty acid which has anti-inflammatory properties. For six weeks, take zinc ascorbate to increase immune resistance and healing of the tissues. • **[BC]**

Reading
Super Skin by Kathryn Marsden, £5.99, Thorsons.

Hints
Four tablespoons of aloe vera juice drunk daily in fresh juice has helped many readers as it helps to heal soft tissue.

A rest often helps alleviate this condition, so take regular holidays. Use washing powders and detergents suitable for sensitive skin. Ultra-violet light often brings relief, but only do this under the supervision of a dermatologist. Moderate amounts of sunshine can help too, but try to avoid direct sunlight between 11am and 3pm.

Chickweed ointment. For details, call 0171 436 5122.

Homeopathy has helped many sufferers (*see* **Useful Information** *for full details*).

LOW BLOOD PRESSURE (Hypotension)

The classic symptom of low blood pressure is light headedness on standing. Low blood pressure is not thought of as a problem in this country by conventional doctors, but in certain European countries it is often treated. Because the blood is responsible for carrying oxygen and nutrients to the body's tissues, low blood pressure can often cause problems with energy and mental function.

Low blood pressure can sometimes be a sign of weakness in the adrenal glands, which sit on top of your kidneys and have an important role to play in our hormonal system. Adrenal weakness is due mainly to dietary deficiencies and stress and is becoming increasingly common. If you know that you have low blood pressure and are continually exhausted, see a doctor who is also a nutritionist and he/she can suggest specific supplements to support adrenal function.

Diet

Nutritional deficiencies can cause the walls of blood vessels to lose elasticity, which become flabby and expand. A high-protein diet which includes organic chicken, fresh fish, lentils, beans, pulses and soya bean curd (tofu) can help restore elasticity to the arteries and help normalize blood pressure. Avoid junk foods like hamburgers and do not eat sugar, which puts the adrenal glands under enormous stress (*see* **General Health Hints**).

167

Supplements
Silica tablets to restore elasticity to the blood vessels. Vitamin E starting at 100–200iu per day for a week or so and working up gradually to 1,000iu daily can help normalize blood pressure. Also take 1g of vitamin C daily, along with a B complex with an additional 500mg of B5 (pantothenic acid) to support adrenal function. Cactus and Hawthorn Complex is a simple herbal remedy that can help low blood pressure. Siberian ginseng can also help normalize low blood pressure. • [BLK]

LOW BLOOD SUGAR (Hypoglycaemia)
The level of sugar in your blood is critical to how you feel. Sugar is the essential fuel in your body and if the blood sugar levels fall, you will feel tired and lethargic. People who have low blood sugar tend to suffer from fluctuating energy as their blood sugar level varies during the day. Another common symptom is to feel very tired on waking, despite getting a decent amount of sleep. Low blood sugar doesn't just affect physical energy, it can sap your mental energy too. The brain uses a lot of the body's sugar supply, and even relatively minor drops in blood sugar can lead to loss of memory and poor concentration. Low blood sugar is also linked with mood disturbances such as anxiety, irritability and depression. It is also associated with cravings for sweet and sometimes starchy foods. Obviously, if your blood sugar level is low, it is natural for your body to ask you to eat the foods it knows will replenish sugar most quickly into the blood stream, such as sweets and chocolates. In the long term, the over-consumption of these foods actually exacerbates this problem. Occasionally, the symptoms of low blood sugar may actually be a sign of diabetes (high blood sugar). Therefore, it is important to see your GP

if you suffer from these symptoms. However, a single blood test is unlikely to show up a problem with low blood sugar because, unless you are actually suffering a dip in blood sugar at the time of the test, the result will be normal.

Diet
The way to treat low blood sugar is to ensure that you maintain a stable level of sugar in the blood throughout the day. It is important to eat regular meals, including breakfast. Many people who suffer from this condition find that it is much more beneficial to eat five or six small meals during the day rather than having just two or three main meals. Another way to do this is to eat fruit or other healthy snacks in the mid-morning and mid-afternoon. It is also essential to cut down on foods which release sugar quickly into the blood such as refined sugar, white bread, white rice, white pasta, shop-bought cakes and pastries. Base your diet around foods which release sugar relatively slowly into the bloodstream such as brown rice, wholewheat pasta, wholemeal bread, fruit, vegetables, meat and fish. Coffee, tea and other stimulants should be avoided, as these tend to cause the blood sugar level to roller-coaster. Herb and fruit teas and coffee substitutes, available in good health food stores, are much healthier.

Supplements
Take a multivitamin/mineral with a B Complex and 3g of vitamin C. The mineral chromium, in which many people are deficient, is vital for balancing blood sugar and reducing sugar cravings. Calcium, magnesium and the amino acid glutamine also reduce cravings because they supply fuel to the brain. Essential Balance Oil provides essential fatty acids (*see* **Fats You Need to Eat**). • **[HN]**

Reading
Low Blood Sugar by Martin L Budd, £7.99, Thorsons.

Recipes For Health: Low Blood Sugar by Maggie Budd-Martin, £6.99, Thorsons.
Diabetes and Hypoglycaemia by Michael Murray, £9.95 Prima Press.

Hints
If you have acute symptoms such as fainting fits, blackouts, extreme weakness and trembling, it is important to restore blood sugar levels as quickly as possible. Although I never recommend that anyone should take refined sugar normally in their diet, this is one situation where something sugary such as a biscuit or soft drink is warranted.

Hypolarm is a perspiration alarm which has a sensor that attaches to the skin. The alarm is used while asleep and a two-tone alarm wakes the user to warn of a dangerously low fall in sugar levels. For further information, contact 0181 441 9641.

Your own GP can refer you to the nearest doctor who is also a qualified nutritionist (*see* **Useful Information** *for further details*).

LOW STOMACH ACID (*see also* **Acid Stomach** *and* **Indigestion**)
Our stomachs secrete hydrochloric acid (HCl) which is essential for the digestion of protein in the diet. As we age, levels of acid often drop, leading to poor digestion of food in the gut. Low stomach acid can lead to poor absorption of nutrients which may give rise to conditions such as osteoporosis.

When stomach acid is low, there is a risk that incompletely digested food can end up leaking into the bloodstream causing food allergies. Also, undigested food can rot in the gut causing bloating, wind and overgrowth of unhealthy organisms like candida. Ironically, many people who have low stomach acid think they have too much, and start taking antacids which can exacerbate the problem in the long term. By supplementing the diet with HCl, along with a digestive enzyme tablet, the situation can often be alleviated.

Diet
Anything which helps digestion is going to help this problem. Chew thoroughly, don't eat too much at one sitting and avoid drinking with meals. Avoid eating too fast and cut down on alcohol and coffee consumption. Food combining is also excellent for this problem as it takes the strain off the digestive system. Meat or fish mix well with vegetables other than potato. Do not mix protein like meat or fish with starches like potatoes, rice or bread. Starchy foods combine well with vegetables, but do not mix any of these with protein (*see* **General Health Hints**).

Supplements
Betaine hydrochloride with pepsin, (but not if you have an active stomach ulcer), along with the enzyme bromelain which aids protein digestion. The healthy bacteria acidophilus can be taken for four weeks to help regulate digestion. • [FSC]

Reading
Food Combining in 30 Days by Kathryn Marsden, £4.99, Thorsons.

Hints
If you have pronounced longitudinal ridges in your nails, this is a common sign of low stomach acid. Drink mint or peppermint herbal teas to aid digestion. Walking for 30 minutes each day (but not immediately after eating) aids digestion. Eat lighter meals when you are upset or stressed

171

as the digestive system does not work properly then.

ME (Myalgia Encephalomyelitis)

ME or chronic fatigue syndrome (CFS) is a condition characterized by long-term incapacitating tiredness and is often also associated with other symptoms such as muscle soreness and depression. The medical profession continues to be divided on whether it is a predominantly physical or mental problem, but there is increasing evidence which suggests that ME is very much a physical illness. Theories abound as to what causes ME; it has been linked to the polio vaccine, but no one explanation has emerged. Possibilities include viral infections, low blood sugar, food intolerance, candida, adrenal exhaustion and nutrient deficiencies (particularly magnesium). Each case is highly individual and sufferers who have written to me find that certain things help one person, but have no effect on another. It is essential to listen to your body and rest as much as possible; over-exertion only exacerbates the problem.

Diet

Avoid all caffeine and alcohol. Reduce intake of sugar-based and pre-packaged foods, which are often high in salt, fat and refined sugar, not to mention artificial additives. Eat plenty of high energy foods like organic fruit, vegetables, wholegrain cereals and quality protein at least twice a day. Cut down on saturated fats, but eat more extra virgin organic olive oil, linseed or walnut oil, which is good for the liver (*see* **Fats You Need to Eat**). Some sufferers have an intolerance to cows' milk, so cut out all dairy products made from cows' milk for a month and see if it makes any difference. Use soya or rice milk and products instead which are non-dairy. Drink plenty of filtered or distilled

172

water, even if you are not thirsty.

Supplements

Oxy-B15 complex (contains vitamin B15, Co Enzyme Q10 and Siberian ginseng) all known to aid energy levels. Magnesium EAP, as magnesium is often deficient in ME patients. B complex to support the nervous system. • **[BC]**

Essential fats are important with ME (*for details, see under* **Fats You Need To Eat**). The herb milk thistle helps detoxify the liver, thereby boosting the immune system. Sublingual B12 for energy and nerves. • **[NC]**

The herb echinacea is a powerful immune booster plus anti-oxidant formula containing vitamins A, C, E plus minerals selenium and zinc. • **[BLK]**

Reading

Chronic Fatigue, Complete Mind & Body Programme by Deepak Chopra, £7.99, Rider.

ME: Post Viral Fatigue Syndrome and How to Live With It by Dr Ann Macintyre, £7.99. From Action for ME; call 0891 122976.

Chronic Fatigue Syndrome by Michael Murray, £9.95, Prima Press.

Hints

Empulse is a pulse electromagnetic treatment, the setting of which is governed by an analysis of the brain's electrical activity. It is a non-invasive, non-drug based preventative treatment. Details are available from: MDI, 17 Owen Road, Diss, Norfolk IP22 3ER or call 01379 644234.

Many people have reported increased energy levels after taking three bee propolis capsules daily for several weeks – for further information on bee propolis, contact: Bee Health Ltd, The Honey Farm, Race Course Road, East Ayton, Scarborough, YO13 9HT or call 01723 864001.

For free dietary advice and an information pack, send an A4 SAE with a 50p stamp to: Action for ME, Department

146, PO Box 1302, Wells, Somerset BA5 2WE. 24-hour information line 0891 122976.

Many readers have literally been cured of ME by a specialist healer called Seka Nikolic and her brother Momo Kovacevic. I know Seka and Momo personally and have interviewed many people (and their doctors), who are now free from ME thanks to Seka and Momo. At the time of going to press, Seka and Momo work from The Hale Clinic, 7 Park Crescent, London W1N 3HE, tel: 0171 631 0156.

Cranial osteopathy or bio-cranial osteopathy has helped many people with ME, as it releases nerve endings which releases energy in the body. With ME, it is best to consult a doctor who is also a qualified nutritionist, as you may need injections of magnesium and B12 (*see* **Useful Information** *for further details*).

MEDITATION

The goal of meditation is to give the brain and, therefore, the entire system a few minutes of total rest each day. When we are active all day our brains generate beta (busy) waves. During the quiet contemplative state induced by meditation, our brains switch to an alpha state. Doctors have proved that people who meditate regularly are less stressful, have stronger immune systems and are generally healthier. Chronic insomniacs find meditation helpful as it assists in learning to shut off the constant 'brain chatter' which keeps them awake. Unfortunately not every health authority recognizes the benefits of meditation, but in certain areas if your GP thinks it would be beneficial, then lessons are available on the NHS. Further information is available from the National Transcendental Meditation Freephone Helpline on 0800 269303 or from Transcendental Meditation, Freepost, London SW1P 4YY.

Reading
Teach Yourself To Meditate by Eric Harrison, £7.99, Piatkus Books.
How To Meditate by Lawrence Leshan, £5.99, Harper Collins.
Available from Watkins Books on 0171 836 2182.

MEMORY (*see also* **Alzheimer's**)

At 47 I often forget why I started a sentence! So to all who have written to me about this problem, don't panic, you are not alone! The brain is like any other organ, it needs nourishment to work efficiently. Low blood sugar is a common cause of poor memory and concentration (*see* **Low Blood Sugar**). The brain also needs oxygen and the fact is that many of us do a pretty poor job of breathing efficiently. Learning a deep breathing technique can also help to spark your brain back into life. Recent research shows that pollutants from household chemicals, drugs, smoke, pesticides, exhaust fumes and industrial pollution all affect the delicate balance of the brain. Avoid exposure to all pollutants as much as possible.

Diet
Diets high in refined carbohydrates can cause blood sugar problems. Avoid shop-bought cakes, biscuits and white bread, which deplete the body of B vitamins. The majority of people with dementia are deficient in vitamin B12 and folic acid. Stimulants like coffee, tea, chocolate and colas all deplete vital nutrients from the body. Eat plenty of brown rice, wholemeal bread and pasta, oat-based cereals, barley, organic vegetables and fruits. If you crave sugar, then use a little organic honey or rice syrup (*see* **General Health Hints**).

Supplements

Brain Food is a supplement especially designed to feed the brain containing niacin(B3), pantothenic acid (B5), phosphatidyl choline, arginine and DMAE (*for further details, see* **Alzheimer's**).

Lecithin granules, which include phosphatidyl choline, are good for memory and circulation; take at least one tablespoon daily. The herb ginkgo biloba is known to improve circulation, especially to the brain, if 60–120mg of standardized extract are taken daily. A digestive enzyme with main meals to aid digestion and absorption of nutrients from food. A multi-vitamin and mineral. For details of all the above supplements and a free leaflet 'Feeding the Brain – Can Nutrients Make us Smarter?', call 01435 882880.

Magnesium taurate together with phosphatidyl serine are extremely important for improving brain function. • **[BC]**

Reading

Smart Nutrients by Dr Abram Hoffer, £9.95, Avery. To order, call 0171 436 5122. Dr Hoffer is a world renowned expert on nutrients for the brain with 30 years in this field.

Toxic Metal Syndrome by Dr H Richard Casdorph/Dr M Walken, £14.20. Explains how memory can be affected by toxins. To order, call 0171 436 5122.

How To Develop A Super Power Memory by Harry Lorayne, £3.99, Thorsons.

Hints

If your memory does not improve within three months of trying these suggestions, see a nutritionist who is also a doctor (*also see* **Alzheimer's** *hints section*).

MENOPAUSE (*see also* **Osteoporosis**)

For women, menopause is a natural part of the ageing process and usually occurs somewhere between the ages of 45 to 55. Menopause is the result of the decline in ovarian function leading to much decreased levels of the hormone oestrogen and a complete cessation of progesterone production. Common symptoms include hot flushes, night sweats, loss of libido, vaginal dryness, palpitations and problems with mood, such as depression and anxiety. I do not advocate taking orthodox hormone replacement therapy (HRT) because of the increased risk of hypertension, weight gain, gall bladder and liver problems, not to mention breast and endometrial (womb) cancers. Orthodox HRT slows the rate of bone density loss, but only while you are taking it.

Diet

Chinese and Japanese women do not suffer with menopausal symptoms as we do in the West. This is because they eat plenty of soya products and fresh vegetables which contain hormone regulating nutrients called isoflavones and phytosterols. We, on the other hand, tend to overload our bodies with synthetic hormones and additives from many of our foods, which have been sprayed with herbicides and pesticides. These compounds like lindane have an oestrogen-like effect. Excess intake of oestrogen, which is the main ingredient in the Pill and HRT, increases the risk of breast and endometrial cancers.

Millions of cattle and chickens are regularly fed with large doses of antibiotics to reduce infection. Animals also eat grasses and feed that are contaminated with pesticides, which then enter our food chain which has an oestrogen effect on the body. These residues accumulate in the fatty tissue of our breasts. Eat organic meat, chickens and vegetables if you want to avoid all these dangerous pollutants. Also eat plenty of foods that help regulate hormone levels like sage, broccoli, cabbage, kale, cauliflower, soya products, alfalfa, celery, beetroot and fennel. Avoid too much caffeine, alcohol, colas and tea (*see* **General Health Hints**).

Supplements

Agnus castus is a traditional European herb commonly used for many menopausal symptoms which can be taken in conjunction with dong quai. These herbs also help with excess hair on the face and body due to the menopause. • **[BLK]**

Vitamin E 200–400iu, taken in combination with ginseng and 50–100mg of vitamin B6, helps ease hot flushes. 2g of vitamin C as magnesium ascorbate, a multi-vitamin especially for women (like Femforte) plus a calcium, magnesium and zinc combination. • **[BC]**

Menophase contains Mexican yam and dong quai, plus all the vitamins and mineral a menopausal woman needs. • **[HN]**

Reading

Balancing Hormones Naturally by Kate Neil, £4.95, ION Press.
Natural Alternatives to HRT by Dr Marilyn Glenville, £9.75 (inc p&p), Lifestyles Press. Available from: Lifestyles Press, 37 High Street, New Town, Uckfield, East Sussex TN22 5DL. Marilyn's book is a must for any woman who wants to handle the menopause naturally through dietary changes and supplements.
What Your Doctor May Not Tell You About Menopause by Dr John Lee, £11.20, Warner (inc p&p) from Natural Progesterone Information Service, BCM Box 4315, London WC1N 3XX.
Natural Progesterone by Dr John Lee, £12.00. Available from ION. To order, call 0181 877 9993.

Hints

Natural progesterone has been available for over 20 years in America and was available here from health stores until the Medicines' Control Agency decided it should be on prescription. It is currently available over the counter from health stores in America and Ireland. In the UK natural progesterone cream is available on prescription. Many gynaecologists and doctors prefer natural progesterone to orthodox HRT. It can be used by women who, for medical reasons, cannot take conventional HRT. As with any hormonal treatment, there are potential hazards with progesterone and it is wise only to use it if you have been shown to really need it. Diagnostech is a specialised laboratory service which offers hormone measurements based on saliva samples. For details, send an SAE to: Diagnostech, The Cottage, Lakeside Centre, 180 Lifford Lane, Kings Norton, Birmingham, B30 3NT.

This supplement must be prescribed by your own GP or you can contact a private doctor who has a knowledge of natural progesterone. If you require further information on natural progesterone and a list of doctors who work with this treatment, send £2 to: Natural Progesterone Information Service, BCM Box 4312, London WC1N 3XX.

Natural progesterone is also available in the form of an oil, cream or tablets which can be placed under the tongue. You can order the oil and cream for your own use from: PharmWest in Ireland, tel: 00 353 1862 1309 and the tablets from PharmWest in the USA, tel: 001 310 822 0823/fax: 001 310 577 0296.

Sylk, a natural lubricant made from kiwi fruit with no additives, is wonderful for easing vaginal dryness. Available from 0181 874 1130.

MERCURY FILLINGS

Over the last few years there has been increasing concern that a significant number of us are being poisoned by the amalgam fillings in our teeth. Research exists showing that mercury can suppress the healthy functioning of our immune system. Many people have found that their chronic health problems have improved after removal of their amalgam fillings. However, this procedure should only be undertaken by a dentist who is skilled in this technique as there is the possibility that mercury can be swallowed or mercury vapour inhaled during the treatment.

Diet
Avoid chewing gum which can increase the level of mercury in your mouth (*see* **General Health Hints**).

Supplements
Supplements which help to de-toxify the body of mercury are 2g of vitamin C as magnesium ascorbate, zinc ascorbate, plus Aminoplex, which contains methionine, cysteine and lysine, amino acids known to aid detoxification of the body. An anti-oxidant formula plus selenium 200mcg daily. • **[BC]**

Reading
Dentistry Without Mercury by Sam and Michael Ziff, £3.95, Probe Inc. To order, call 0171 436 5122.
BioMed Report on Amalgam Toxicity by Dr Alan Hibberd, 65p plus first class stamp from BioMed Publications, 16 Court Oak Grove, Harborne, Birmingham.

Hints
For specialist help in the removal of amalgam fillings, contact Jack Levenson, a leading dentist who specializes in this field. The Brompton Dental Clinic, 221 Old Brompton Road, London SW5 0EA. Tel: 0171 370 0055. A fact sheet, *Poisons in The Mouth,* is available from this address.

There is also a specialist blood test which shows up metal toxicity. For further details, contact: The British Society for Mercury Free Dentistry, 1 Welbeck House, 62 Welbeck Street, London W1M 7HB.

MIGRAINE

Migraines are usually one-sided headaches which can be preceded by some form of visual disturbance such as flashing lights or partial blindness. The severity of the attack can vary enormously, ranging from a relatively mild attack lasting a few hours, to a very severe headache with nausea and vomiting lasting several days.

Diet

Avoid the foods known to trigger migraine attacks; especially cheese, red wine, chocolate, coffee, wheat and citrus fruits. Toxaemia, especially in the bowel, can result in headaches, as certain bacteria in the colon can convert tyrosine to tyramine which is thought to trigger attacks in many sufferers. If you tend to be on the constipated side, take raw organic linseeds and plenty of water as this will help to reduce toxicity in the bowel (*see* **Constipation**). Skipping meals is another trigger for migraine and this may well relate to problems with low blood sugar (*see also* **Low Blood Sugar** *and* **General Health Hints**).

Supplements

3g of evening primrose oil daily. The ingredients are thought to block inflammatory compounds which are involved in causing migraines. Healthy bacteria like acidophilus between meals to keep the bowels clean. Magnesium 200–400mg, as a deficiency is often associated with migraine. Take a digestive enzyme complex to help digestion which reduces the likelihood of allergic reaction to undigested food particles. • **[LGF]**

Reading
The Natural Way With Migraine by Eileen Herzberg, £3.99, Element Books.
Migraine Revolution by Dr John Mansfield, £4.99, Thorsons.
Migraine Handbook by Jenny Lewis, £6.99, Vermilion Press.
TMJ – The Jaw Connection by Greg Goddard, £11.50, Aurora.

Hints
Migraine is often triggered by food allergies, so keep a food diary to see if you can identify foods that cause an attack. If this is unsuccessful, a consultation with a qualified kinesiologist is well worthwhile. Regular aerobic exercise has been shown to reduce migraine attacks and yoga helps reduce stress levels.

Many readers have found that grinding their teeth over many years often causes the jaw to slip out of alignment. This causes blood flow to the head to be restricted, bringing on regular headaches like migraines. If you see a dentist who specializes in TMJ (Temporo-Mandibular Joint Syndrome), they can make a small brace to be worn at night to hold the jaw in the correct position which often alleviates all symptoms. To find a practitioner, send an SAE to: The Cranio Group, Wretham Lodge, Priory Road, Forest Row, East Sussex RH18 5HR. Also many migraine sufferers have problems with vertebrae in their neck which disrupt blood flow to the brain. See a chiropractor or a cranial osteopath who can re-align the neck and head (*see* **Useful Information** *for details*).

Many people have found that by wearing magnetic jewellery pain is relieved. For further details and a brochure, send an SAE to: Acar-Sud, Westfield House, Hampton Court Road, East Molesey, Surrey KT8 9BX. Tel: 0181 877 1699.

Further information can be obtained from the British Migraine Association on 01932 352 468. Send a large SAE to: 178a High Road, Byfleet, West Byfleet, Surrey KT14 7ED.

Empulse is a pulsed electromagnetic treatment, the setting of which is governed by an analysis of the brain's electrical activity. It is a non-invasive, non-drug based preventative treatment. Further details are available from: MDI Ltd, 17 Owen Road, Diss, Norfolk IP22 3ER or call 01379 644234

MOUTH PROBLEMS

Mouth Problems – Burning Mouth Syndrome

Symptoms include tongue swelling, metallic tastes and a burning sensation in the mouth. Nitrates and added chemicals found in drinking water can cause this syndrome, so try using a nitrate removing water filter or install a good quality water filter like Watersimple from The Fresh Water Filter Company – for further details, call 0181 558 7495. Avoid toothpaste and tooth powders which contain additives, aluminium and chemicals like fluoride. Use a herbal toothpaste like Blackmores, Sarakan or aloe vera.

Supplements
A deficiency of vitamin B12 can also cause these symptoms, so take a good multi-vitamin daily which includes B12, as well as a multi-mineral supplement containing zinc. Also take two acidophilus capsules daily to re-balance your whole digestive system. • [BLK]

Hints
Mouth problems often reflect problems in the gut and

183

digestive system. See a nutritionist who can re-balance your diet and suggest supplements to boost your immune system (*see* **General Health Hints**).

Mouth Problems – Cracked Lips

Lips that are cracked and sore at the corners of the mouth usually denote a deficiency in the B vitamins, especially B2. Dry cracking lips are associated with a lack of vitamin E and essential fatty acids found in oils such as evening primrose oil or walnut oil. Also include more extra virgin olive oil in your everyday diet.

Supplements
A multi-B complex plus vitamin C, also 200iu of vitamin E and 1,500mg of evening primrose oil daily which eases the dryness in your skin. Many women are also deficient in zinc, which is essential if wounds are to heal. Take 30mg daily for six weeks and rub vitamin E cream onto the affected area.

Hints
Use a lip balm like Lobello every day to help keep the lips moisturised.

Mouth Problems – Mouth Ulcers

Recurring mouth ulcers can be linked to nutritional deficiencies, especially zinc and B vitamins, and often occur when the immune system is low or when foods are eaten to which you have an allergic reaction. Many readers have found oranges and tomatoes are a problem, whilst others found that ill-fitting dentures bring on an attack.

Diet
Avoid any products containing sugar or white flour. Also

avoid nuts (especially peanuts), strawberries, tomatoes, pineapple and any highly acidic fruit such as plums, rhubarb, kiwi fruit and citrus fruits (*see* **General Health Hints** *below*).

Supplements
Take a multi-vitamin/mineral, 1g of vitamin C, zinc ascorbate, liquid vitamin A one drop daily in juice, which is easily absorbed and aids soft tissue healing, until the bottle is finished. • **[BC]**

Vitamin B Complex plus 400mcg of folic acid for recurrent mouth ulcers. Stop taking the folic acid once ulcers have cleared but continue with the B complex.

Hints
Tea tree oil is a natural antiseptic and makes a marvellous mouthwash when a few drops are mixed with warm water. Some readers have found that they are allergic to the material that false teeth are made from. Ask your dentist to test you for an allergy – use porcelain as an alternative material as this has been found to ease the discomfort. Pierce a vitamin E capsule and apply the oil to the ulcers. I find that if I use toothpaste containing fluoride I get mouth ulcers. Try and avoid all fluoride.

MULTIPLE SCLEROSIS – MS
Multiple sclerosis is a progressive disease affecting the nervous system. It often develops over many years during which time the patient experiences attacks of weakness, visual problems or loss of sensation in certain parts of the body. Attacks are normally interspersed with periods of recovery, but each attack will normally leave some lasting symptoms. The rate at which the condition progresses

varies considerably from person to person.

Dr Patrick Kingsley, one of the UK's most experienced nutritional physicians dealing with MS, states that in his opinion mercury is a very important factor in multiple sclerosis, as he has found that many of his patients have an average of 7.5 times more mercury in their spinal fluid than a healthy person should have. Dr Kingsley has found that severe candida yeast infection sometimes mimic MS symptoms and are often mistaken for MS (*see* **Candida**). Food sensitivities can also play a role in MS.

Diet

Avoid foods high in saturated fat, red meat, cows' milk, cheese, pastries, snacks, yeast and wheat. Replace wheat with rye breads and rice or oat cakes. Increase your intake of essential fatty acids found in evening primrose oil and fish oils. Eat plenty of pumpkin, sunflower seeds and linseeds which are also rich in essential fatty acids. Eat wholegrain cereals, like brown rice, barley, buckwheat, quinoa and organic fruit and vegetables, especially greens and use extra virgin olive oil in dressings (*see* **General Health Hints**).

Supplements

Certain supplements aid elimination of mercury but according to Dr Kingsley this can take up to nine months after the mercury fillings have been removed (*see* **Mercury Fillings** *for these supplements*). Try a regime that includes supplements known to de-toxify the body such as liquid selenium, 2g of vitamin C daily, plus 30mg of zinc plus a multi-mineral, magnesium EAP, reduced glutathione, 400–800iu vitamin E and a B complex. Essential fatty acids are vital for people with MS (*see* **Fats You Need to Eat**).

Dr Kingsley has found that patients who have sensory problems like pins and needles and numbness often benefit from vitamin B12 injections (5–6mg). He says this treatment is definitely worth trying.

Reading
Multiple Sclerosis by Judy Graham, £9.99, Thorsons.
The Natural Way with Multiple Sclerosis by Richard Thomas, £3.99, Element Books.
Diets to Help Multiple Sclerosis by Rita Greer, £3.99, Thorsons.

Hints
People on vegan or gluten-free diets often have relief from symptoms – but the diet would need to be kept up for at least two years, because vegan diets are rich in essential fats needed for nerve function and low in saturated fat.

There is a yoga centre which specializes in helping MS patients to recover mobility and self-confidence. For details, send a large SAE to: Yoga For Health Foundation, Ickwell Bury, Near Biggleswade, Bedfordshire SG18 9EF. Tel: 01767 627 271.

Help and advice on MS can be obtained from Solent Multiple Sclerosis Therapy Centres on 01705 699116. Send an SAE to 56 Hewitt Road, Portsmouth PO2 OQP.

NAIL PROBLEMS

Nail Problems – Fungal Infections

Fungal infections usually cause discoloration and deformity in affected nails. This problem is more likely to occur when your immune system is not functioning properly.

Diet
Avoid all junk food and any products containing sugar for at least four weeks, as these lower the immune system and

slow the healing process. Also avoid foods containing yeast such as bread, alcohol, soy sauce, Marmite, Bovril, mushrooms and vinegar. Try eating yeast-free soda bread (*see* **General Health Hints**).

Supplements
Dab tea tree oil, which is naturally antiseptic and anti-fungal, directly onto the nails. In a recent study it was found that 92% of women in the UK are deficient in zinc, which is essential for healing and to strengthen the immune system. Take 30mg daily for six weeks. 2g of vitamin C plus echinacea herbal tablets make an excellent immune system booster. • **[FSC]**

Take two acidophilus capsules daily for six weeks to help replenish the good bacteria in the gut which are destroyed by fungal infections.

Nail Problems – Splitting and White Spots

Diet
Iron deficiency is a common cause of nail problems (*see* **Anaemia**). To increase iron intake, include plenty of fresh fish, poultry and green leafy vegetables in the diet. As vitamin C increases iron absorption, include plenty of fruit in the diet whilst avoiding coffee and tea with a meal as these prevent iron being absorbed. Eat plenty of raw or lightly cooked, yellow and orange vegetables. Incorporate plenty of extra virgin olive oil and live yoghurt in your diet.

Supplements
White spots in the nails are usually a sign that you are low in the mineral zinc. If your nails are brittle or splitting, take a calcium, magnesium and zinc complex for three months. • **[S]**

This can also be caused by poor absorption of nutrients

from food. Take a digestive enzyme daily along with a multi-mineral, plus essential fatty acids like linseed oil. • [FSC]

Hints
Massage olive oil or evening primrose oil regularly into the nails and cuticles which speeds the growth of nail tissue.

NUMB AND TINGLING SENSATIONS, Fingers and Toes
This may be a sign of sluggish circulation. Extremes of cold can cause numbness and tingling, as during cold weather circulation to the skin is reduced (*see* **Circulation**). Any conditions which reduce the circulation to nerves in the skin will produce a similar sensation.

Diet
A deficiency of essential fatty acids found in linseed oil, sunflower seeds, borage oil and oily fish can cause this problem. Eat plenty of red and purple fruits like bilberries, blueberries and cherries which are high in flavonoids to help strengthen capillaries (*see* **General Health Hints**).

Supplements
Take three teaspoons of organic linseed oil on salads or vegetables and a quarter teaspoon of sublingual (under your tongue) vitamin B12 every day, as lack of B12, especially in older people, is known to cause tingling. A multi-vitamin plus a B complex to help support nerves. Sprinkle one tablespoon of lecithin granules on your breakfast to help repair nerve endings. 2g of vitamin C with bioflavonoids daily to aid circulation and repair small capillaries. • [HN].

Hints

If after taking these supplements for six weeks, you still have numb and tingling fingers or toes, see your GP. Walking for half an hour each day will help to get your circulation moving. It is also helpful to massage your hands and feet. Obviously it is easy to massage one's own hands, however if you find it difficult to massage your feet, ask your partner, relative or friend to do it for you. Reflexology and acupuncture often help this type of problem (*see* **Useful Information** *for further details*).

OSTEO-ARTHRITIS (*see* **Arthritis**)

OSTEOPOROSIS (*see also* **Low Stomach Acid** *and* **Menopause**)

Osteoporosis is a condition in which the bones become thin and weak, and prone to fracture, particularly in the hip and spine. The condition is more common in women than in men and usually occurs after the menopause when hormones which help keep bones strong are lost. Women who are very thin and those who smoke are most at risk. Osteoporosis is also associated with a lack of exercise, excess protein in the diet, stress, low weight, low calcium consumption, fizzy drinks and steroids.

Traditionally, osteoporosis is prevented and treated with hormone replacement therapy (HRT). A study in the *New England Journal of Medicine* stated 'Women who have taken HRT for ten years or more may have a greater bone density than those who have not taken it, but lose increased density rapidly when the HRT is stopped and end up with only

3.2% higher bone density than women who took nothing. HRT can only prevent osteoporosis if it is taken for the rest of these womens' lives.'

The work of Dr John Lee in the USA suggests that women who use natural sources of progesterone can increase their bone density quite dramatically, without having to endure the potential side-effects of conventional HRT. Natural progesterone in the form of a cream absorbed through the skin, is available on prescription in the UK. It can increase bone density therefore reducing the risk of osteoporosis at any age. It can be taken instead of conventional HRT (*for full details, see* **Menopause**.)

Diet

Western diets are mainly based on acid-forming foods like proteins and carbohydrates which force the body to compensate by withdrawing calcium from the bones to alkalize the system. According to a Harvard study we eat on average 50% too much protein, especially animal protein which can lead to calcium loss. Vegetarians who eat lots of pulses, beans and lentils for protein suffer less incidence of osteoporosis. Coffee, tea, fizzy drinks and all acid-forming foods leach calcium from the bones, so to maintain a balance, eat plenty of fresh organic vegetables, fruit, broccoli, kale and seaweed which alkalize the body. For calcium, eat plenty of green leafy vegetables, fish and sesame seeds, rather than dairy products made from cows' milk, which are high in saturated fat. Use non-dairy rice or soya milk. Silica found in lettuce, celery, millet, oats and parsnips helps with bone regeneration. Kelp and alfalfa help prevent bone loss (*see* **General Health Hints**).

Supplements

Magnesium is vital to prevent osteoporosis, so take OsteoFormula, a supplement formulated by Dr Alan Gaby containing all the supplements which support bones, such as calcium, magnesium, zinc, vitamin D, vitamin K, vitamin C, manganese, boron, copper, silica and betaine. • **[FSC]**

Take a daily chlorella or green food supplement to keep the body alkalized, along with bamboo gum capsules which are packed with silica, known to stimulate synthesis of collagen in the bone and to help build cartilage. • **[S]**

Reading
Balancing Hormones Naturally by Kate Neil, £4.95, ION Press.
Osteoporosis Prevention and Reversal by Dr Alan Gaby, £17.99, Prima Press.
Osteoporosis by Kathleen May, £4.99, Thorsons.
Natural Alternatives to HRT by Dr Marilyn Glenville, £9.75 (inc p&p), Lifestyles Press. Available from: Lifestyles Press, 37 High Street, New Town, Uckfield, East Sussex TN22 5DL.

Hints
Daylight is needed to make vitamin D in the body, which is essential for absorption and utilization of calcium. For the sake of your bones, make sure that you take some outdoor exercise on a regular basis. Smoking can induce an early menopause and reduce bone mass. Give up for your health's sake. All aerobic and impact exercises like skipping can increase bone density. Also weight-bearing exercises help to strengthen bones. Regular exercise of any description is vital to help fight osteoporosis.

For further information on osteoporosis contact: Life Foundation School of Therapeutics, Maristowe House, Dover Street, Bilston, West Midlands WV14 6AL or call 01902 409164.

PALPITATIONS (*see also* **Tachycardia**)
Palpitations can take many forms such as the feeling of the

heart racing, skipped beats or a fluttering in the chest. Normally palpitations are not a sign that anything is seriously wrong with the heart, but occasionally they are due to some problem with the electrical circuitry in the heart. **If you suffer from any of these symptoms – see your GP.**

Diet
Avoid all stimulants in the diet, especially caffeine in tea, coffee, caffeinated soft drinks and chocolate. Food additives can trigger palpitations, so eat a good, clean, unprocessed diet. Alcohol is another common trigger for palpitations, minimize the amount you drink or eliminate it completely (*see* **General Health Hints**).

Supplements
Co-enzyme Q10, 30–60mg each day, known to regularize the heart beat. Vitamin B complex helps the heart to beat regularly. Irregular heartbeat is often linked to calcium/magnesium imbalance or deficiency. Take a magnesium, calcium and zinc formula to support nerves, muscles and the heart.

Hints
If you feel an attack beginning, splash your face with cold water and lay down for a few minutes until the feeling passes. Learn to meditate which reduces stress, as worrying about this condition can precipitate an attack.

PANIC ATTACKS
Panic attacks are a very common problem affecting an estimated ten million people in Britain alone. Along with a feeling of intense panic, sufferers tend to breathe very

quickly (hyperventilation) which can produce feelings of light headedness and tingling in the fingers and toes caused by too much oxygen. Sometimes, panic attacks are triggered by a traumatic life event such as the death of a close one or loss of a job. Panic attacks can be linked to low blood sugar which will tend to make sufferers feel tense and nervous (*see* **Low Blood Sugar**).

Diet
Keeping the blood sugar level even is essential for combating panic attacks. Make sure you eat regularly throughout the day and don't skip meals. Stick to foods that release sugar relatively slowly into the blood stream including fruits, vegetables, unrefined starches such as brown rice and wholemeal bread, meats and fish (*see* **General Health Hints**).

Supplements
Vitamin B complex daily helps reduce stress. NT188 contains B vitamins and passiflora to keep you calm, plus magnesium to support nerves. 1g of vitamin C. Chromium polynicotinate is excellent for stabilizing blood sugar levels. • [BC]

There is a supplement containing kava kava root, from the South Pacific. When taken regularly it has the cumulative effect of relaxing the body and banishing anxiety. • [S]

Reading
Panic Attacks by Christine Ingram, £5.99, Thorsons.
The Power is Within You by Louise Hay, £8.99, Eden Grove Editions.
Stress Control Through Self-Hypnosis by Dr Arthur Jackson, £7.99, Piatkus Books.
Anxiety, Phobias and Panic Attacks by Elaine Sheehan, £4.99, Element Books.

Hints

Avoid caffeine, sugar and alcohol which can cause severe mood swings and may disrupt blood sugar levels.

Bach Flower remedies are helpful for panic attacks. Regular exercise reduces stress and builds confidence. A regular aromatherapy message helps you to stay calm. A warm relaxing bath and sound, restful sleep does wonders to ease stress. Learn how to control the attacks; fighting them will only make them worse. Tell yourself that this is just the body's way of getting you to take care of yourself. Speak to yourself gently, as you would to comfort a child.

The Phobic Society, 4 Cheltenham Road, Chorlton-cum-Hardy M21 9QN. Tel: 0161 881 1937, is a registered charity to help with anxiety disorders, teaching self-help rather than drug related therapies. Send an SAE for further information.

First Steps to Freedom is a self-help group. For further information, call their helpline on 01926 851608.

PARKINSON'S DISEASE

This is a progressive disorder of the nervous system resulting from degeneration of brain cells. Parkinson's commonly begins with a tremor in one limb. Movement becomes progressively more difficult and simple tasks can become a nightmare. Lack of the brain chemical dopamine makes the condition worse and most sufferers take a synthetic form of the amino acid L-Dopa to help restore brain function. Many of the drugs associated with Parkinson's cause lethargy and extreme mental confusion. **I strongly suggest that anyone diagnosed with Parkinson's should *immediately* consult a doctor who is also a nutritionist, as this condition needs very specialist care.**

What works for one person may be useless to another and many highly specialist amino acids are needed in specific doses to suit the individual case.

Diet

Dr Melvyn Werbach, who is a well-known authority on nutritional influences on disease, says that restricting intake of protein is helpful and that 90% of the daily intake of protein should be eaten with the evening meal. Eat no more than 0.8g of protein for each kilogram of body weight. Eat plenty of high-fibre foods to avoid constipation. Fresh broad beans contain levodopa, known to help treat Parkinson's. Eat daily when in season (*see* **General Health Hints**).

Supplements

Parkinson's has been linked to low levels of B6, folic acid and niacin, all of which are B vitamins. Try taking a B complex for six months and see if symptoms improve. Take at least 3g of vitamin C daily, along with 400iu of natural vitamin E. As anti-oxidants have been helpful to many people, take an anti-oxidant formula plus a multi-mineral and a multi-vitamin. Essential fatty acids are vital for brain function; take a 1g linseed oil capsule daily. Co-enzyme Q10 has helped many sufferers; take 60mg daily. A co-enzyme, known as NADH, is essential for the L-Dopa to be effective. Some studies using NADH have shown promising results, such as reduced disability. For further information on this supplement, call 01435 882 880.

Reading

Parkinson's Disease, The Nutritional Handbook by Dr Geoffrey Leader and Lucille Leader, £10. Available from The Chronic Pain Relief and Nutritional Support Clinic, Devonshire Hospital, 29 Devonshire Street, London W1N 1RF.
Parkinson's Disease by Dr Abraham Lieberman & Frank Williams, £8.99, Thorsons.

Hints

Aluminium and mercury have been linked to Parkinson's, therefore avoid all aluminium cookware and don't use aluminium foil. For more details of mercury, *see* **Mercury Fillings**. As many of the world's oceans are heavily polluted, high levels of mercury are also being reported in fish. Monosodium glutamate (MSG), the food additive, has been linked to Parkinson's; therefore avoid all additives and preservatives whenever possible. Use a good quality water filter like Watersimple from The Fresh Water Filter Company. Further details are available from 0181 558 7495. This water purifier will help to reduce the amount of heavy metals and chemicals in drinking water. As organo-phosphates (OPs) are now found in drinking water, many sufferers find some relief when they switch to purer water (*see* **General Health Hints**).

PHLEBITIS

Phlebitis is caused by inflammation of the walls of the veins and produces red, tender veins. Phlebitis is often associated with the formation of small blood clots on the areas of inflammation, giving rise to a condition known as thrombophlebitis. Phlebitis is more common if blood should tend to stagnate in the veins such as when the veins are varicose. The best way to prevent this condition (or to manage further episodes) is with a combination of regular gentle exercise and good nutrition.

Diet

Include plenty of oily fish like salmon and mackerel in your diet. Cut out saturated fats found in red meat, cheese, full cream cows' milk and chocolate. Eat more foods containing essential fats like cold pressed organic walnut, sunflower oil, nuts and seeds. Use organic olive oil, high in vitamin E, for salad dressings and try Vitaquell spread instead of butter. Eat plenty of fresh fruit and vegetables and include wholemeal bread, pasta, brown rice and oats in your diet. Use rice milk and try sheeps' or goats' yoghurt. Add fresh garlic to main meals as it helps to thin the blood (*see* **General Health Hints**).

Supplements
Take an anti-oxidant formula containing vitamins A, C, E, and the minerals selenium and zinc. Bromelain is a natural digestive enzyme extracted from pineapples which is good for phlebitis – take with main meals. • **[S]**

Flax seed oil helps to thin the blood. Add it to salads or vegetables or drink one tablespoon in juice daily (*see* **Fats You Need to Eat**). • **[HN]**

Reading
Optimum Nutrition by Patrick Holford, £5.95, ION Press.

Hints
Exercise may be painful initially and should only be undertaken after discussion with your doctor. Begin by walking for 30 minutes each day increasing to one hour after six weeks. Swimming, yoga or Qigong, an extremely gentle and easy exercise regime, would also be helpful, as would reflexology (*see* **Useful Information** *for details*).

PHOBIAS
Many readers have written in with phobias of varying kinds. Some have a chronic fear of spiders, while others have been afraid to leave their homes for years. Whilst many people find this type of condition hard to understand,

the person with the phobia is truly living a nightmare. Counselling for the whole family may be necessary.

Diet
Avoid eating too many stimulants like sugar, alcohol, coffee and tea which can cause severe mood swings adding to your problem (*see also* **General Health Hints** *and* **Low Blood Sugar**).

Reading
Stress Control Through Self-Hypnosis by Dr Arthur Jackson, £7.99, Piatkus Books.
Self-Hypnosis by Valerie Austin, £5.99, Thorsons.
Paul McKenna makes excellent self hypnosis tapes. For details, contact: Paul McKenna Associates on 01455 852233.

Hints
First Steps to Freedom, a self-help group with a helpline 365 days a year for people with phobias. Counselling, tapes and leaflets are available. The membership fee is £7.50 per year. For further information write to First Steps to Freedom, 22 Randall Road, Kenilworth, Warwickshire or call 01926 851608.

Hypnotherapy is an excellent way to find the root cause of your problem and learn how to let it go in order to lead a normal life (*see* **Useful Information** *for further details*).

PILES – HAEMORRHOIDS (*see also* **Constipation**)
Piles are the result of veins just inside the anus becoming enlarged. Generally, piles remain inside the anus, but can sometimes protrude externally and may even get stuck in this position requiring immediate medical attention. Piles can give rise to pain, bleeding and itching in the anal area.

Piles tend to run in families and they can be precipitated by pregnancy, prolonged periods of sitting or standing and constipation.

Diet
Keep your diet rich in fibre to prevent constipation, which is a common factor in piles. Eat plenty of fresh fruits and vegetables and wholegrains like brown rice, wholemeal bread and pasta, oats and barley. Drink at least eight glasses of filtered water daily, which is also essential for regular bowel function. Additional healthy fibre can be obtained by adding agents such as linseeds or psyllium fibre to your diet. Avoid meat, which slows up bowel movement as it takes a long time to digest (*see* **General Health Hints**).

Supplements
Primarily avoid constipation; take at least one tablespoon daily of a soluble fibre like organic linseeds to keep the bowels regular. Take 2g of vitamin C with bioflavonoids and the herb gotu kola helps to heal the delicate skin tissue in the bowel. Grape seed extract 100–300mg a day which helps to protect skin tissue, is a natural antibiotic and helps to keep the bowels regular. • **[FSC]**

Hints
Calendula and vitamin E cream applied topically will reduce soreness.

PILL – The Contraceptive Pill
The progesterone only, or mini-pill, provides contraception by thickening the mucus in the cervix and making it impenetrable to sperm. The combined pill, which contains both oestrogen and progesterone, prevents pregnancy by

suppressing ovulation. The Pill is associated with a number of potential hazards and side-effects including an increased risk of cancers of the breast and cervix, blood clots in the legs (deep vein thrombosis), high blood pressure, increased risk of heart disease and stroke, weight gain, fluid retention and migraine.

Diet
The Pill can deplete many nutrients in the body such as zinc, iron, B group vitamins especially B6, B12 and folic acid, vitamin C, magnesium and calcium. These nutrient deficiencies, combined with stress and an unbalanced diet, will have a noticeable long-term affect on the immune system and can cause depression. Eat a diet high in wholegrains like brown rice, wholemeal bread, pulses and lentils. Raw wheatgerm is high in vitamins B and E. Organic fruits and vegetables are high in natural carotenes, vitamin C and other nutrients (*see* **General Health Hints**).

Supplements
A good multi-vitamin/mineral. 15–30mg of zinc ideally to be taken last thing at night for maximum absorption and 1g of vitamin C daily.

Reading
Optimum Nutrition by Patrick Holford, £5.95, ION Press.

Hints
There are many natural methods of contraception including the rhythm method and barrier methods, which are healthier than the Pill. For further details, contact the Natural Family Planning Centre, Birmingham Maternity Hospital, QE Medical Centre, Birmingham B15 2TG. If you are on the pill you should not smoke, as this considerably increases the risk of some hazards such as blood clots and heart disease.

PMT/PMS – Pre-Menstrual Tension/Pre-Menstrual Syndrome

PMS is characterized by a collection of potentially distressing symptoms prior to menstruation. These symptoms can be mood-related, such as depression, irritability and fearfulness, or they may be more physically orientated such as breast tenderness, fluid retention, food cravings and abdominal bloating. Low blood sugar is common prior to the start of menstruation and can contribute to the mood problems and the food cravings (*see* **Low Blood Sugar**). PMS is also associated with low levels of progesterone and excess oestrogen (*see* **Menopause** *for details of a natural progesterone supplement which may be of benefit in severe cases of PMS*).

Diet

Medical studies have shown that a diet low in fat, sugar, salt and dairy foods made from cows' milk may reduce symptoms. Use soya or rice milk and products which are non-dairy. Excess sugar can cause anxiety, irritability and depression. Cut down on caffeine and alcohol, drink herbal teas and sugar-free drinks. Low levels of the hormone serotonin have been linked to PMS. This hormone helps us to feel more positive and, by eating unrefined carbohydrates, serotonin levels are increased naturally. Eat a diet high in foods which release their sugars slowly into the bloodstream and raise serotonin levels, like oats, brown rice, brown pasta and bread and barley. Include plenty of organic fruit and vegetables in your diet. Eat small healthy meals regularly which helps to balance blood sugar levels (*see* **General Health Hints**).

Supplements

These supplements should be taken every day, not just

around the time of your period: a multi-vitamin for women such as Femforte, Mega GLA; an essential fatty acid often deficient in PMS which helps to relieve breast tenderness and period pains; B6 100mg. At least 1g of Vitamin C as magnesium ascorbate plus 200iu of vitamin E daily. PT208 containing agnus castus, a herb known to help PMT. Bio-magnesium, as magnesium deficiency is linked to PMS. • [BC]

Take Siberian Ginseng if you are exhausted as the ginseng supports adrenal function (avoid if you have high blood pressure).

Reading
The Pre-Menstrual Syndrome by Caroline Shreeve, £4.99, Thorsons.
Beat PMT Through Diet by Maryon Stewart, £6.99, Headline. To order call 0181 877 9993.
The Natural Way With PMS by Jane Sullivan, £3.99, Element Books.

Hints
When you are stressed, you produce too much adrenalin which eventually exhausts your endocrine (hormone) system. Start taking more regular exercise to reduce stress or learn to meditate. Find some time each day to call your own even if it's only a relaxing bath for 30 minutes. Treat yourself to an aromatherapy massage each month. Many women with PMS also have *Candida* (*see* **Candida** *for further information*).

POST-NATAL DEPRESSION
The birth of a child is usually a time of unparalleled happiness and joy. Yet, for some women, childbirth can

herald a down-swing in mood which is termed post-natal depression. The condition is poorly understood and conventional medicine usually has only anti-depressants and tranquillizers to offer.

Diet
It is essential that the diet is kept healthy during this time as pregnancy and childbirth (not to mention breast-feeding) put enormous strain on the body. The diet should be full of fruits, vegetables and wholegrains, with as little sugar, saturated fat and processed foods as possible (*see* **General Health Hints**).

Supplements
Post-natal depression is associated with low levels of B vitamins and minerals like calcium, magnesium and zinc, which should all be taken for at least two months.

Positive Nutrition is a special formula for depressed people with the amino acids glutamine and tyrosine, and vitamins and minerals like B3, B6, magnesium and zinc which are all needed to metabolize the amino acids. Also a multi-vitamin plus 3g of vitamin C a day. • **[HN]**

Reading
Alternative Maternity by Nicky Wesson, £8.99, Vermilion.

Hints
Post-natal depression is often caused by the sudden fall in progesterone levels just before birth in women whose bodies are slow to begin making progesterone again. Pro-Gest is a natural progesterone cream which is easily absorbed and will bring your progesterone level up again until your body takes over. For further details and a list of doctors who work with natural progesterone, send £2 to: Natural Progesterone Information Service, BCM 4315, London WC1N 3XX.

* ❋ *

PRICKLY HEAT

Prickly heat is characterized by a rash of tiny inflamed pimples that come up in the sun, which often itch quite severely. Suffers of prickly heat often have underlying food sensitivities that sensitize the skin, making it more likely to respond to heat (*see* **Allergies**). Certain antibiotics are also known to cause this problem.

Diet

Try cutting out cows' milk, wheat, peanuts and coffee, although the culprits could be something quite unusual like radishes, bananas or orange juice. Detoxify your body as much as possible by drinking lots of water and eating plenty of fresh vegetables and fruit (*see* **General Health Hints**).

Supplements

Take 2g of vitamin C with bioflavonoids (which act as a natural antihistamine). Two tablespoons of organic flax seed oil, which is rich in essential fats to feed the skin, on your vegetables or salad every day plus a multi-vitamin/mineral. • **[HN]**

Natural carotenes are known to nourish the skin and may help to avoid sun-related skin rashes if taken regularly. Take a carotenoid complex derived from natural sources. • **[S]**

Reading

Allergy and Intolerance by G Lewith, £9.99, Green Print. Available from Green Library on 0171 385 0012.

Hints

Many strong antibiotics and drugs make the skin very sun-sensitive. If you are taking antibiotics, stay out of the sun. Often emulsifiers and chemicals in sunscreens can cause prickly heat. I use Soltan or Vichy for really sensitive skins from Boots. Stay out of the midday sun and never allow your skin to go red. Use unperfumed bath soaps and gels when on holiday. Many readers report relief from prickly heat after using concentrated aloe vera gel on the skin both under their sunscreens and applied after sun bathing. The homeopathic remedy *sol30* has helped many people to prevent and heal prickly heat – but it is not a substitute for sun block. For details, call 0171 935 5330.

PROSTATE

The prostate is a walnut-sized gland that sits below the bladder in the male. The tube that takes urine from the bladder to the outside (the urethra) passes through the prostate. As men age, the prostate can enlarge, so impeding the flow of urine from the bladder. Common symptoms include difficulty in starting urination, poor stream, frequent urination, often with the need to get up at night and dribbling after the end of urination. The majority of prostate problems are due to a condition called benign prostatic hypertrophy (BPH), but occasionally the prostate can be affected by cancer. **Prostate problems are becoming more common in younger men and if you feel you have a prostate problem, it is *VITAL* for you to see your doctor immediately so that your condition can be properly assessed and treated quickly.**

Diet

Reduce your intake of high fat dairy products made from cows' milk, eat plenty of fresh chicken and fish. Try to eat organic foods – as new research shows a link between pesticide residues and prostate enlargement. Studies show that an enlarged prostate is often linked to a zinc deficiency, eat lots of pumpkin seeds which are rich in zinc and essential fatty acids. Eat plenty of fibre, oat bran and cereals, linseeds, fruit and vegetables. Japanese men eat a diet that is rich in soy beans, tofu and vegetables like broccoli and cauliflower which contain plant oestrogens known to have a protective effect on the prostate (*see also* **General Health Hints**).

Supplements

1g of linseed oil and Formula 600 containing zinc, saw palmetto, African pygeum and amino acids, which are all helpful for prostate conditions. • **[FSC]**

Anti-oxidant nutrients such as vitamins A, C, E, a natural carotene complex and the minerals zinc and selenium have been shown in many scientific studies to inhibit cancer cell growth. All men from the age of twenty onwards should take a good quality anti-oxidant formulation.

Reading

Prostate Cancer by Philip Dunn, £7.99. To order from the Prostate Help Association, Langworth, Lincoln LN3 5DF.
Prostate Problems: The Complete Guide by Jeremy Hamand, £7.99, Thorsons.
The Complete Book Of Men's Health by Dr Sarah Brewer, £9.99, Thorsons.

Hints

To help improve circulation to the area and reduce inflammation, lie on your back, bend your knees, bring the soles of the feet together and bring the feet as close to your buttocks as possible. Relax your legs, letting the knees fall outwards towards the ground. Hold this position for five minutes. Only attempt this exercise if you are fit and have no joint problems in your hips and legs.

Many men have reported that taking a supplement called Prost8 has helped with benign prostatic hyperplasia (BPH). Includes bee pollen, glycine, vitamin B6, ginseng, zinc gluconate, vitamin E and beta carotene. For further details of Prost8 call Natural Health Supplements on 01243 771700 or send an SAE to: Natural Health, 1st Floor, Victoria Court, St Pancras, Chichester, West Sussex PO19 4LT.

See an osteopath or chiropractor to check that the pelvis and spine are not misaligned, as in certain cases a major nerve connection from the lower part of the spine to the prostate becomes trapped and once this is released water can be passed normally (*see* **Useful Information** *for further details of this*).

For further help and advice, send a large SAE to: The Prostate Help Association, Langworth, Lincoln LN3 5DF or Prostate Research Campaign UK, 36 The Drive, Northwood, Middlesex HA6 1HP.

PSORIASIS

Psoriasis is a chronic skin condition characterized by patches of red, raised, scaly skin. There does seem to be some hereditary link in psoriasis, but often symptoms may not appear until adulthood. The severity of the condition can vary enormously from person to person and time to time. Many doctors feel that stress triggers this condition, so any relaxation exercise like yoga or meditation may help.

Diet

Cut out all animal fats and alcohol, and eat oily fish like salmon, mackerel, sardines, tuna and herrings, as well as plenty of fresh fruits and vegetables. A diet low in refined sugar and citrus fruits is advised. It is vital to make sure that you have enough essential fats in your diet, therefore take at least one tablespoon of pure cold pressed linseed oil every day (*see also* **Fats You Need To Eat** *and* **General Health Hints**).

Supplements

Liquid vitamin A, one drop (equal to 5,000iu of vitamin A) daily in juice to help heal the skin. 1g linseed oil capsules, 2g of vitamin C with bioflavonoids and NutriGuard Forte (a powerful anti-oxidant containing beta carotene, lycopene, vitamins A, C, E and selenium), plus 30mg of zinc citrate, as zinc is vital in healing skin. Vitamin C cream can be applied topically (do not apply to broken skin). • **[BC]**

Milk thistle is marvellous for liver cleansing and clearing the skin. Take daily for two months. • **[BLK]**

Reading

Super Skin by Kathryn Marsden, £5.99, Thorsons.
Beat Psoriasis by Sandra Gibbons, £7.99, Thorsons.
Aloe Vera – The Legendary Healer by Alasdair Barcroft, £6.99, Souvenir Press. Available from 0181 871 5083.

Hints

Some doctors are now treating their patients successfully with aloe vera juice. Take two tablespoons of this daily in fresh juice.

Cherryfields Clinic specializes in herbal remedies which can be taken internally and used externally. Their preparations have had excellent results. For further information contact the Hale Clinic on 0171 631 0156.

Sea bathing is beneficial for psoriasis. Many sufferers find relief after bathing in Dead Sea salt because of its high mineral contents. Add 2lb to your bath and soak for ten minutes. Moderate sun exposure also helps psoriasis, but remember to wear a hypoallergenic sun screen.

RAYNAUD'S DISEASE

Raynaud's is an intermittent spasm of the small arteries in

the fingers and toes, usually associated with exposure to cold. The digits turn white and numb and then, as they warm up, they become red and usually painful, depending on the severity of the spasm. Sometimes the skin can actually ulcerate if it is starved of blood for too long.

Diet

Ensure an adequate intake of iron from lean red meat, poultry, fish, leafy green vegetables (especially broccoli) and complex carbohydrates like brown rice, barley, potatoes, wholemeal bread, pasta, oat-based cereals and seeds. Avoid drinking tea and coffee as this inhibits iron absorption, as does smoking. Include plenty of sunflower, pumpkin and linseeds in the diet, which are high in essential fatty acids (*see also* **Fats You Need to Eat** *and* **General Health Hints**).

Supplements

Ginkgo Plus contains the herbs ginkgo biloba and bilberry. Potassium ascorbate, a form of vitamin C to aid circulation. Mega GLA is a vital essential fatty acid known to aid this condition, take two capsules daily. 60mg of Co Enzyme Q10.

200–400mg of magnesium and 100iu of natural vitamin E to improve circulation, a multi-mineral containing manganese to support the nervous system. • **[BC]**

In some severe cases, injections of vitamin B especially B12 have proved helpful. Take a B complex daily along with a sublingual (dissolved under the tongue) form of vitamin B12. • **[NC]**

Hints

Take regular exercise to improve circulation. Swimming, skipping and re-bounding on a mini-trampoline are all wonderful ways to improve circulation. I suffer from this condition as a result of varicose vein surgery. I was told that

I had plenty of veins left, but it has reduced my circulation drastically. If you are thinking of having veins removed, you might like to keep this in mind. Wear warm socks for most of the year in bed. Never wear tight-fitting shoes which restrict circulation.

Also try wearing magnet insoles in your shoes, which aid circulation. Nikken UK, Unit 7, Landmere Lane, Edwalton, Nottingham NG12 4DE.

Try massaging hands and toes regularly with diluted oil of black pepper and rosemary. Reflexology and acupuncture have helped many sufferers (*see* **Useful Information** *for further details*).

For further information and advice contact: The Raynaud's and Scleroderma Association, 112 Crewe Road, Alsager, Cheshire ST7 2JA.

REPETITIVE STRAIN INJURY – RSI
Anyone who has a job which involves repetitive movements is at risk from problems with their finger, hands, wrists or arms. Most sufferers of RSI spend a substantial part of their day sitting in front of a VDU or typewriter. Symptoms are usually worse if their sitting posture is incorrect.

Diet
(*see* **General Health Hints**.)

Supplements
2g of vitamin C as magnesium ascorbate to help reduce inflammation. Ligazyme (containing calcium, vitamin C, bromelain and magnesium), plus Colleginase (containing rutin, silica, vitamins A and D) to support connective tissue, maintain strong bones and aid healing. B Complex plus

211

100–200mg of B6 for six weeks. • **[BC]**

Reading
Are You Sitting Comfortably by Andrew Wilson, £6.99, Optima. Available from Green Farm Library on 0181 874 1130.
RSI–Repetitive Strain Injury by Wendy Chalmers Mill, £3.99, Thorsons.

Hints
Magnets can help relieve localized pain. For details, send an SAE to: Acar-Sud Distribution, Westfield House, Hampton Court Road, East Molesey, Surrey KT8 9BX or MagnePlast, Welbeck House, 63 Wellington Road, Pinner, Middlesex HA5 4NF.

Derma C Cream. Massage in after a warm shower, cover with cloth to avoid staining clothes until absorbed. • **[BC]**

If your work involves long hours at a computer screen, then the Ergo Rest will place your arm in the right position helping to reduce muscle fatigue and pain in the neck. For further details, send a large SAE to Incoms Systems, Rowan House, 9–31 Victoria Road, Park Royal, London NW10 6DP. Tel: 0181 838 0077.

The Alexander Technique helps individuals learn about healthy posture and therefore, how to reduce or even eliminate RSI problems. Acute problems may benefit from treatment with osteopathy, chiropractic or acupuncture (*see* **Useful Information** *for further details*).

RESTLESS LEGS
Also known as Ekbom's Syndrome, this condition is characterized by aching, tickling, burning or twitching in the muscles of the legs. It occurs particularly at night or when

sitting still for long periods. Restless Legs is often related to cramps at night and is thought to be due at least in part to poor circulation to the legs. It is particularly common in pregnant and middle-aged women, smokers and those who drink lots of caffeine. It is also commonly found in people who are deficient in iron, vitamin E and magnesium.

Diet
Avoid all caffeine containing drinks like cola, tea and coffee and do not eat late at night. Eat a diet rich in nuts, seeds, avocado, green leafy vegetables, fish and poultry. Smoking is not advisable (*see* **General Health Hints**).

Supplements
Try an iron formula like Spatone which includes vitamins B and C, which are vital for iron absorption – from good health stores. Vitamin E 200iu daily, 200mg of magnesium plus Mega GLA, an essential fatty acid that helps circulation and is anti-inflammatory. A multi-vitamin/mineral plus a B complex, along with Ginkgo Plus containing the herbs ginkgo biloba and bilberry is known to improve circulation. • [BC]

Hints
A simple blood test will tell you if you are anaemic and actually need to take extra iron (*see* **Anaemia**). Get plenty of exercise. Massage your legs and feet using kneading movements from the ankle upwards towards the knee. The legs can be bathed in alternate hot and cold water to improve circulation. Try reflexology, acupuncture or regular aromatherapy massage to pep up the circulation. Take all the suggested supplements above for at least three months.

RHEUMATOID ARTHRITIS (*see* Arthritis)

ROSACEA

Rosacea is characterized by a red rash which usually affects the skin around the nose. Rosacea can be inherited or related to emotional stress, tension, menopause, climatic conditions such as bright sunshine or certain foods and drink, especially alcohol, tea, coffee and spicy foods. There is evidence to suggest that up to 90% of sufferers do not make enough stomach acid and incomplete digestion of food is the true underlying cause of this condition.

Diet

Avoid junk and sugar-based foods, as well as dairy products made from cows' milk and cheese. Use goats', sheeps', soya or rice milk, yoghurt and cheese instead. Eat plenty of fresh fruit and vegetables. Drink at least six glasses of filtered water every day. Avoid coffee, tea, colas, alcohol, very hot drinks and spicy foods that often cause flushing. Research indicates the tremendous benefits of eating raw organic vegetables regularly; particularly cabbage, broccoli, cauliflower and spinach; or blend these into a vegetable juice cocktail. These vegetables contain chemicals which help modulate hormone levels and improve the liver's detoxification function.

Supplements

Take at least 1g of vitamin C with bioflavonoids, which strengthens the tiny blood vessels in the skin. Plus a B complex daily, as sufferers are often low in B vitamins. Betaine hydrochloride, stomach acid. **(Do not take Hydrochloric Acid supplements or a digestive enzyme if you have active stomach ulcers).**

Acidophilus daily on an empty stomach to replenish good bacteria in the gut, plus a liquid gel multi-vitamin capsule which is easily absorbed. • **[FSC]**

Reading
Super Skin by Kathryn Marsden, £5.99, Thorsons.

Hints
There is a skin regime called Sher which has helped many sufferers. For full details, contact The Sher System, 30 New Bond Street, London W1Y 9HD. Tel 0171 499 4022.

SAD SYNDROME – Seasonal Affective Disorder

SAD syndrome is a condition in which sufferers complain of depression or low mood during the winter months when lack of sunlight can have an important affect on the biochemistry in the brain leading to low mood, lack of energy or depression. During the winter we produce less of the hormone melatonin. In summer, thanks to natural sunlight, we make more melatonin, the hormone which helps enhance our mood. It is a well-established fact that the suicide rates rise in Scandinavian countries during the winter months.

Supplements
To support your nerves and reduce stress, take NT188, a high potency vitamin B complex containing herbs like passiflora which help nerves, plus 100–200mg of magnesium. • **[BC]**

Positive Nutrition is a special formula for depressed people with the amino acids glutamine and tyrosine plus vitamins like B3 and B6, and the mineral magnesium needed to utilize the amino acids in the body. • **[HN]**

Taking 3mg of melatonin each night can help relieve symptoms. This is available on prescription from your GP; call 0171 436 5122 for further details.

Reading
Day Light Robbery by Dr Damien Downing, £3.99, Arrow Books.
SAD by Angela Smyth, £5.99, Thorsons.

Hints
Exercise as much as possible during daylight which will reduce feelings of depression by stimulating production of melatonin. Spectra light is a special portable lamp which gives out a full spectrum of natural daylight and can be used for up to one hour daily to alleviate SAD syndrome. For further details, call 0171 631 0156.

Contact the SAD Association who have a support network, by sending a large SAE to: PO Box 989, London SW7 2PZ.

SCALP PROBLEMS

Scalp Problems – Dry, Flaking, Itching Scalp

Many people have this problem and I note that the majority are over 50. From listening to their dietary regime it appears that this problem is nearly always linked to a lack of essential fats (*see* **Fats You Need to Eat**). It can also be linked to eczema or psoriasis. Also a common cause of an itchy scalp and dandruff is candida (*see* **Candida**).

Diet
Eat more oily fish like salmon and mackerel and use olive

oil, walnut oil or organic sunflower oil for salad dressings. **Never** fry or cook with these oils. Stop using all refined mass-produced oils, which have virtually no nutritional value and, once heated, become dangerous. Eat more fresh fruits and vegetables and avoid too many saturated fats and sugar in the diet (*see* **General Health Hints**).

Supplements
A good quality multi-vitamin and mineral every day. 1g linseed oil capsule daily, plus 200iu of vitamin E.

Hints
Use natural-based shampoos that contain no chemicals and colourings. Massage the scalp with a natural antiseptic like tea tree oil lotion. Blackmores make an excellent range, available from all good health stores. Massage scalp with jojoba oil and leave on overnight.

Scalp Problems – Greasy Scalp

This problem seems more common in men and can be linked to hormonal changes.

Diet
Cut all saturated fats – especially red meats – from the diet as these putrefy in the gut. Regular head massage and exercise will help reduce the amount of sebum you are producing. Drink at least six glasses of filtered or distilled water every day. Include more soya products in your diet, plus plenty of fresh vegetables like broccoli and cauliflower which regulate hormones (*see* **General Health Hints**).

Supplements
Herbs like saw palmetto and sarsaparillo help to detoxify the body, heal skin and balance male hormones naturally. • **[S]**

A multi-mineral containing zinc (which is often lacking) plus a multi-vitamin, 2g of vitamin C daily and Mega GLA (an essential fatty acid). • [BC]

Reading
Natural Solution to Hair Loss and Scalp Problems by David Satchell, £5.50. Available to order from 01323 645164.

Hints
Consult a qualified nutritionist who can help you to re-balance your diet (*see* **Useful Information** *for further details of this service*).

SCIATICA
Sciatica is usually a symptom of a structural problem in the lower back, where the nerve is pinched as it emerges from the spinal column. Classically, sciatica gives rise to pain which runs down the back of the leg, often as far down as the knee and sometimes down to the foot. The pain is sometimes accompanied by numbness or tingling.

Diet
Avoid coffee which inhibits the body's ability to cope with pain (*see* **General Health Hints**).

Supplements
NT188 contains vitamin B and passiflora to calm the nerves, plus 250mg of magnesium malate twice daily to relax nerve endings. 2g of vitamin C daily, which has an anti-inflammatory effect, as does Mega GLA, an essential fatty acid which helps to reduce inflammation. • [BC]

DLPA is an amino acid which helps the body deal with pain. • [LGF]

218

Ginger and turmeric capsules are often more effective than some steroids for pain relief. Take four daily while symptoms are severe. • [FSC]

Hints
When sleeping or resting, lie on your side with a pillow between your knees to minimize pelvic strain.

To reduce pain and discomfort, prepare an icepack and a hot water bottle wrapped in a towel. Place each alternatively on the site of the pain for ten minutes and repeat; this should be done twice daily.

Many alternative practitioners have found that regular deep tissue massage gives enormous relief to sciatica sufferers as often muscular pain in this area can be mistaken for sciatica. There is a special type of massage called tuina which has proved extremely beneficial. For further details of a practitioner in your area, send an SAE to: Body Harmonics Centre, 54 Flecker's Drive, Hatherley, Cheltenham GL51 5BD.

Try osteopathy, a chiropractor or acupuncture for further relief (*see* **Useful Information** *for further details*).

SHINGLES
Anyone who has had chickenpox will still have the virus lying dormant in their body. Even if you do not remember having chickenpox as a child, you can only suffer shingles once you have had chickenpox. In certain circumstances, the virus can reactivate, giving rise to a painful, red rash, usually on one side of the chest. Because the virus is normally kept in check by the immune system, it is when the immune system is at a low ebb that shingles will tend to occur, when we are stressed, exhausted or overworked.

Diet

Increase daily intake of vitamin C rich foods, such as fresh fruit, vegetables, parsley, kiwi fruit and strawberries as vitamin C helps to boost the immune system and is a potent anti-viral agent. Avoid chocolate, carob and nuts which worsen the condition because they contain an amino acid, which can encourage growth of the virus. Avoid all refined carbohydrates like white bread, shop-bought cakes, biscuits and soft drinks, which are often high in sugar and can dampen the effectiveness of the immune system (*see* **General Health Hints**).

Supplements

Liquid vitamin A (one drop equals 5,000iu of vitamin A), one drop daily in juice to aid skin healing, plus GLA, an essential fatty acid. A multi-vitamin/mineral plus 2g of vitamin C to boost the immune system, 300iu vitamin E. • **[BC]**

The amino acid lysine can be very effective in stopping shingles in its tracks because it disrupts the replication of the virus. Take 2g of lysine, plus 2g extra of vitamin C every day whilst the attack lasts.

The herb hypericum, commonly known as St John's Wort, has proved helpful for the itching and lingering pain associated with shingles, as it is anti-viral and helps soothe nerve endings which are often irritated. The herb echinacea helps to boost the immune system and milk thistle helps detoxify the liver. • **[BLK]**

Liquorice applied topically and taken internally can also help kill the virus. • **[FSC]**

Reading

Super Skin by Kathryn Marsden, £5.99, Thorsons.

Hints

Vitamin E oil capsules pierced and applied to the sores may give some relief. Vitamin B12 injections on a regular basis have helped many people. Hypericum and comfrey oil can also be massaged in to the affected areas to bring relief.

SINUS PROBLEMS (*see* **Allergic Rhinitis, Allergies** *and* **Catarrh**)

SLEEPING PILLS , ADDICTION (*see also* **Insomnia**)
The big problem with sleeping pills is that they can lead to addiction in the long term. Also, there is always the risk that the medication may make the insomnia worse by disturbing the delicate chemical balance of the brain, which is essential for it to function normally. To avoid withdrawal symptoms, see your GP, who can advise you on how to gradually reduce the dose.

Natural remedies may not work for the first two weeks due to the toxic residue in your liver left over from the drugs. Remember it takes at least one month to kick the habit of addiction, so be patient.

Supplements
Take a detoxifying agent like the herb milk thistle, available in capsules or tincture form, or dandelion tea with plenty of water to help cleanse the liver, for at least six weeks. Also drink fresh vegetable juices, especially beetroot which is very cleansing. Recent research in America has found that niacinamide (vitamin B3) helps to ease anxiety and in some cases relieves insomnia. Because the benzodiazepine family of sleeping pills replicate the action of niacinamide (a naturally occurring nutrient in the brain), this substance helps induce sleep. Try taking 500–1,000mg of B3, 45

221

minutes before retiring. Make sure that you take a B complex with breakfast to help support the nerves. Also take a calcium, magnesium and zinc complex as these minerals are often deficient in people who wake during the night. • **[FSC]**

Positive Nutrition is an amino acid formula which helps you to get over addiction to sleeping pills (*see* **Depression** *for further details*).

Reading
They Said I Was Dead by Anne McManus. A personal story of how to cope and come through addiction. Available from Scarlet Press, 5 Montague Road, London E8 2HN, £8.99.
Stress, Anxiety and Insomnia by Michael Murray ND, £9.95, Prima Press.

Hints
For over 20 years I have had a problem sleeping, but find that when I am on holiday I sleep like a log. Most of us today lead very stressful lives and have a lot on our minds and at night our brains seem to wake up. If this is your problem, I strongly suggest you learn to meditate and include more regular exercise which reduces stress. Take a natural herbal remedy like Formula Z, which is derived from valerian and wild lettuce, herbs proved to aid restful sleep and relaxation. For details, call 01204 707420. Bioforce also make an excellent tincture called Dormesan containing hops, lemon balm and valerian which have sedative properties. Useful for people who tend to wake during the early hours. There are literally dozens of natural sleep remedies – ask for advice at your local health store.

SMOKING

If you smoke, then the biggest single contribution you can make to your future health is to stop. Smoking doesn't just increase your risk of a variety of cancers, heart disease and stroke, it also speeds up the ageing process in the body through the production of enormous amounts of free radical molecules. Studies have shown that the skin of a 40-year-old who smokes is comparable with a 65-year-old non-smoker, so help yourself stay young and give up smoking!

It is imperative that you make a firm resolution that you actually want to stop smoking. Telephone helplines for smokers who need support: England 0171 487 3000; Scotland 0800 848484; Wales 0345 697500; Northern Ireland 01232 663281.

Diet

Eat lots of green vegetables especially broccoli, cabbage and kale. Nearly all fruits and vegetables are rich in natural beta carotenes which help to reduce the risk of developing certain cancers (*see* **General Health Hints**).

Supplements

For smokers and passive smokers it is vital to ensure a regular intake of the anti-oxidant nutrients beta-carotene, vitamins A, C and E, plus the minerals zinc and selenium. Vitamin B is also essential for the nervous system, which can be damaged by smoke inhalation. Try Natural Flow's mega multi daily which includes all these vitamins. • **[LGF]**

It is also important to take 100–200mg niacin (vitamin B3), also called nicotinic acid, which helps to reduce nicotine withdrawal.

Reading

Stop Smoking For Good by Robert Brynin, £4.99, Hodder and Stoughton.
The Easy Way To Stop Smoking by Allen Carr, £6.99, Penguin.

Hints

Traditional Herbals make a Smoker's Tea to help people through a nicotine craving. Made from crushed lobelia leaves, which Mexican Indians used to chew as a tobacco substitute, the tea is available from health stores, or by mail-order from Wild Oats in London on 0171 229 1063, or try nicotine patches from all good pharmacies.

The medical herbalist Andrew Chevallier suggests this remedy. Mix one heaped teaspoon of coltsfoot and half a teaspoon of thyme into a teapot of boiling water, cool and sip. Coltsfoot strengthens the lungs and thyme is antiseptic and healing. For details, call Neal's Yard Remedies on 01865 245436.

SORE THROATS (*see also* **Colds and Flu**)

Sore throats are often caused by infection but can also be caused by toxicity in the body, especially when the immune system is low. Infections are normally caused by a bacteria and/or a virus. Antibiotics have no effect on viral infections, but are often prescribed anyway. If the sore throat is chronic and you have tried antibiotics, which help for a short time before the throat becomes sore again, then you urgently need to boost your immune system. Repeated antibiotics will lower the entire immune system. Antibiotics often wipe out the good gut bacteria in the gut, which can lead to all sorts of problems including overgrowth of yeast (candida) and digestive problems.

Diet

Reduce dairy products made from cows' milk and all meats. Try rice milk, which is low in fat for a few weeks. Avoid all products which increase mucus production, such as white bread, shop-bought cakes, chocolate and all foods containing white refined sugar. Eat lots of fresh vegetables, especially carrots and other yellow vegetables, which are high in the anti-oxidant beta-carotene. Soup made from fresh garlic, onion and fresh ginger in a miso stock base should help relieve a sore throat when sipped throughout the day.

Supplements
Chloride compound (200mg) helps to clear lymphatic congestion and can relieve sore throats. While symptoms are severe, take one tablet every four hours. A duo formula containing the herb echinacea and vitamin C, called Echinacea A C E, helps reduce the severity and duration of a sore throat, as both agents boost the immune system, if taken for at least three months. You will also need to repopulate your digestive system with friendly bacteria that will have been killed off by the antibiotics, so take four acidophilus bifidus capsules daily for six weeks after taking any antibiotics. • [BLK]

Take a good multi-mineral vitamin supplement and suck zinc gluconate lozenges, to relieve the sore throat. The herb goldenseal is excellent as it has antibacterial qualities, along with echinacea which boosts the immune system. Solgar make a formula which includes both these herbs, plus cat's claw which is a highly anti-inflammatory plant extract. Take nine capsules daily until the throat soreness eases.

Hints
The herb thyme is a natural antiseptic, and can be made into a solution and used as a gargle for sore throats or sipped as a tea mixture to help relieve sore throats and coughs. Bee Propolis throat spray and lozenges also help relieve a sore throat. Tea tree oil is a natural antiseptic, use diluted with a little sea salt as a gargle, but do not swallow. Homeopathic *belladonna* is also good for sore throats.

STITCH

A stitch is abdominal pain or discomfort that comes on when we exercise and goes away when we rest. It is sometimes possible to exercise through a stitch – but it's rather painful! The pain from a stitch is almost certainly caused by a spasm in the intestinal wall. A sedentary lifestyle, eating too few green vegetables and including too much sugar, caffeine and animal protein in the diet causes a reduction of calcium and magnesium in the body, leading to a build-up of lactic acid which can result in regular attacks of muscle cramps or stitch.

Diet
Include plenty of broccoli and dark green cabbage, spinach and kale in your diet. Make sure you drink at least six glasses of water daily (*see* **General Health Hints**).

Supplements
A calcium/magnesium supplement to alleviate the muscle cramps. • **[FSC]**

Reading
Optimum Nutrition by Patrick Holford, £5.95, ION Press.

Hints
A stitch is more likely to occur if you exercise while food is still digesting in the gut. Avoid exercise for about three hours after a substantial amount of food. Take regular exercise to avoid acid accumulation in the body.

STOMACH AND DUODENAL ULCERS *see also*
Acid Stomach

Ulcers can occur in the stomach, but are more commonly found in the duodenum, which is the part of the intestinal tract just after the stomach. Generally, ulcers cause pain and discomfort and are often associated with a burning sensation felt in the middle of the abdomen, just underneath the ribs.

Ulcers seem to be linked to stress, but it is likely that food sensitivities and problems with digestion are more common underlying causes (*see also* **Acid Stomach** *and* **Low Stomach Acid**). Research in the last few years has found that a bacterium called helicobacter pylori (H. pylori) is present in 90% of cases duodenal ulcers and 80% of gastric ulcers, though it is still not clear how the bug actually causes the ulcer.

Diet

Avoid alcohol, coffee, saturated fats and aspirin, as well as dairy products made from cows' milk. Use non-dairy soya or rice products instead which are low in fat and sugar. Also avoid all foods that contain sugar – this includes sugar-based drinks. Ideally, try drinking a litre of cabbage juice every day, rich in L Glutamine which has been shown to heal peptic ulcers. Cooked plantain bananas are known to give relief. Regular intake of manuka honey from tea tree blossom is anti-bacterial and aids ulcers – one tablespoon daily on an empty stomach before breakfast and dinner. For details, call 0181 961 4410. Eat organic low-fat, live goats' or sheeps' yoghurt (*see* **General Health Hints**).

Supplements

Citricidal, extracted from grapefruit seeds, also helps to kill bacteria and acts as a natural antibiotic. Use up to ten drops in juice daily, it tastes rather bitter, but is often effective. Boost your immune system with anti-oxidant formulas containing vitamins A, C and E, plus the minerals zinc and selenium. Take one tablespoon of organic linseed oil, rich in essential fatty acids (*see* **Fats You Need to Eat**). Healthy bacteria like acidophilus for two months to help heal the gut. The amino acid glutamine heals the digestive lining of ulceration and creates an environment that discourages helicobacter. Aloe Gold, aloe vera juice that is high in mucopolysaccharides to soothe the gut, can be taken before every meal. • **[HN]**

Liquorice taken prior to meals can also help. • **[FSC]**

Reading
Self Help for Stomach Ulcers by Dr Leonard Mervyn, £3.99, Thorsons.
How to Improve Your Digestion and Absorption by Chris Scarfe, £2.50, ION Press.

Hints
Chew food thoroughly. Never rush a meal as digestion is made difficult when you are stressed or in a hurry. Don't drink too much with meals as this dilutes digestive juices. Avoid stress and rushing as much as possible as stress over a prolonged period can cause great harm to our digestive system.

STRESS
Whilst a certain amount of stress is actually good for us, long-term stress can trigger nearly all the major illnesses. When we are stressed, we produce too much adrenalin which, in turn, makes our hearts beat faster, thickens the blood, raises blood pressure. Stress can be the underlying cause of low libido, depression, anxiety, poor digestion, hair loss, eczema, irritable bowel and a whole host of other problems.

Diet

Avoid stimulants like coffee, tea, alcohol, colas, sugar and chocolate. Sugar-based junk foods lower the immune system and deplete energy levels. Keep to a healthy diet which includes plenty of live food like fruit and vegetables which give you more energy. Don't eat late at night; especially heavy or rich foods like red meat or creamy sauces which can take a long time to digest. You are better off eating carbohydrates such as wholemeal pasta, brown rice or barley at night as these have a more calming effect. Low blood sugar can affect your moods and leave you stressed; therefore eat small healthy meals regularly and don't skip meals (*see* **Low Blood Sugar** *and* **General Health Hints**).

Supplements

Take 200–600mg of magnesium a day as stress lowers magnesium levels, plus high potency B tablets, 2g of vitamin C daily, to help boost the immune system. A multi-vitamin/mineral capsule plus an anti-oxidant formula containing vitamins C, E, A, beta carotene, plus the minerals zinc and selenium. Siberian ginseng and 500mg of pantothenic acid (B5) to support adrenal function which is often exhausted when we are under stressed. • **[FSC]**

Kava kava root from the South pacific taken regularly for three months, one hour before bed, helps to give a feeling of calm. • **[HN]**

Reading

How to Stop Worrying and Start Living by Dale Carnegie, £6.99, Mandarin.
Self-help For Your Nerves by Dr Claire Weekes, £4.99, Thorsons.
Teach Yourself To Meditate by Eric Harrison, £7.99, Piatkus Books.
The Duty Trap by Vera Peiffer, £7.99, Element Books.

Hints

Sit back and take time to think – as often you will find that what you most resist is what you most need in your life. You should always try and make a space and some time between what stresses you and your reaction to it. Think about this. Concentrate on what you can change in your life; let go of the things you have no control over. Nearly every one of us suffers stress but it's how we *react* to the stressful situation that's important, as believe it or not we all have choices! Get plenty of exercise which reduces stress. Take yoga lessons and learn how to breathe properly which really does help to reduce stress. Lying down, take a deep breath into your stomach (place your hand on your tummy and actually feel the breath going into the abdomen as it rises) to a count of ten and slowly breathe out to a count of six.

Try a self-help tape called 'Stress Reduction Workshop For Women' by Jacquelyn Ferguson. This is a four-hour workshop on how to cope with stress in everyday life. It teaches relaxation techniques and how to face problems as they arise. For details, call Career Track on 01908 354000. Paul McKenna makes excellent relaxation tapes. For details, contact: Paul McKenna Associates on 01455 852233.

Hypnotherapy, aromatherapy, massage and meditation are all beneficial for relieving stress (*see* **Useful Information** *for further details*).

STROKES (*see also* **Angina** *and* **Heart Disease**)

The brain, like every other part of the body, needs blood to function properly, supplied by arteries. As we age, arteries gradually narrow due to the build-up of fatty cholesterol-like substances. Eventually, an artery may block off altogether leading to the death of part of the brain. This is a stroke. Sometimes a stroke occurs because a blood vessel to the brain bursts, rather than becomes blocked. Usually strokes produce some degree of paralysis down one side of the body, often accompanied by problems with speech. The risk factors for strokes are the same as those for heart disease. Smoking, high cholesterol, high blood pressure, lack of physical exercise and being overweight are the main risk factors. The most important risk factor for stroke is actually high blood pressure.

Diet
Keep your diet as low in salt as possible, as this has been proven to help reduce blood pressure and the risk of stroke. Eat oily fish at least once a week and include plenty of linseeds and pumpkin seeds in the diet, which are high in essential fats. Do not add salt during cooking or at the table and avoid processed foods which have a lot of added salt. Also avoid saturated fats, caffeine and all fried foods. The diet should be full of wholegrains, fruits and vegetables, which are rich in anti-oxidant nutrients such as the vitamins A, C, E, beta carotene and magnesium, which help reduce risk of stroke (*see* **General Health Hints** *and* **The Fats You Need to Eat**).

Supplements
To reduce the chance of strokes, take Lysine C, a combination of lysine and vitamin C, which helps remove the furring of arteries and lessens the risk of having a stroke or heart attack. • **[HN]**

The herb ginkgo biloba improves circulation in the capillaries in the brain, while inhibiting excessive blood clotting. Take 60–100mg of standardized extract daily. Advanced Proanthocyanidin complex (contains pycnogenol, grape seed extract and bilberry extract); all flavonoids known to strengthen capillaries. Take an anti-oxidant complex (containing vitamins C and E, carotenoids, selenium and zinc) as anti-oxidants protect against vascular damage. • [S]

Hints
Many doctors have found that anyone who has suffered a stroke caused by a clot in the brain, should be given intravenous magnesium as soon as possible after the stroke. Magnesium has a powerful dilatory action on the arteries and helps to restore blood flow to the damaged brain tissue. Research shows that people living in soft water areas are more prone to high blood pressure, which can lead to strokes, as soft water is low in magnesium; therefore, if you live in an area of soft water, take a magnesium supplement.

SWOLLEN FEET/ANKLES (*see* **Foot Problems** *and* **Water Retention**)

TACHYCARDIA – RAPID HEART BEAT (*see also* **Palpitations**)
Tachycardia, a sudden increase in the heart rate, is often accompanied by breathlessness, nausea, sweating and dizziness. This condition should always be checked by a doctor.

Diet
Avoid stimulants like tea, coffee, chocolate, colas, alcohol and tobacco, which can bring on an attack of palpitations in people who are sensitive. Low blood sugar can trigger an attack (*see* **Low Blood Sugar**). Eat small, regular meals which include pasta, potatoes, brown rice, barley,

wholemeal bread, vegetables and fruit (*see* **General Health Hints**).

Supplements

Magnesium and vitamin B have a vital role in keeping the heartbeat regular and nourishing the nervous system. Take a B complex along with 200–400mg of magnesium daily. Co-enzyme Q10 30–60mg, has a beneficial effect on the heart. • **[NC]**

Reading

Heart Disease by Richard Thomas, £3.99, Element Books.

Hints

To combat worrying, which only exacerbates the condition, learn how to breathe properly by taking yoga lessons. Also try meditation which teaches you how to stay calm when stressed. If you feel an attack beginning, splash your face with cold water, then lie down, close your eyes, breathe deeply and slowly for a few minutes until the attack passes. Essential oil of lavender has a calming effect, so try a few drops in your bath. Try regular aromatherapy massage, which is very calming. Go for leisurely walks, breathing deeply. The digestive system shuts down when the body is under stress, so avoid eating heavy meals if you are upset.

TASTE AND SMELL, Loss Of

Loss of taste and smell occurs frequently during upper respiratory infections or nasal congestion associated with the common cold (*see* **Catarrh**). This condition can also be caused by a lack of minerals in the body, especially zinc. Certain heart drugs cause loss of taste and smell as a side-effect, so if you are taking heart medication, check with your GP.

Diet

Avoid all mucus-forming foods like cows' milk, cheese, chocolate, red meat, butter, white bread, cakes and biscuits. Introduce more fruit and fresh vegetables into your diet to boost the immune system. Garlic is very cleansing and antiseptic. Eat pumpkin and sunflower seeds which are high in zinc (*see* **General Health Hints**).

Supplements

Histazyme which includes vitamin C and zinc, a lack of which often causes this problem. Also reduces inflammatory response to allergens and protects against infection. • [BC]

Take a good anti-oxidant formula, a multi-vitamin and a multi-mineral to help boost the immune system.

Hints

Tap water is often contaminated by chemicals; invest in a good water filter system like Watersimple. Further details are available from The Fresh Water Filter Company, Carlton House, Aylmer Road, London E11 3AD or call 0181 558 7495.

See a qualified nutritionist who will help to re- balance and de-toxify your system. Homeopathy is also very useful for this particular condition (*see* **Useful Information** *for further details*).

THROAT PROBLEMS (*see* Sore Throat)

THRUSH (*see* Cystitis *and* Candida)

THYROID, Underactive and Overactive

The thyroid gland produces a hormone called thyroxine which controls the rate of metabolism in the body. If the thyroid is overactive and produces too much thyroxine (hyperthyroidism), this causes symptoms such as intolerance to heat, anxiety, palpitations, sweating, loss of weight, bulging eyes, diarrhoea and menstrual disorders.

If the thyroid is underactive and produces too little thyroxine (hypothyroidism) the entire body slows down, causing symptoms such as an intolerance to cold, tiredness, mental sluggishness, weight gain, exhaustion, headaches, constipation, hair loss and coarsening of the skin. It is possible that food sensitivities play a part in this process. One in ten women suffer thyroid problems; if you have any of these symptoms, check with your doctor.

Diet

Poor digestion and absorption, an unhealthy diet and toxins from chemicals such as pesticides and food additives could all contribute a major part in disrupting immune function which may then cause thyroid problems. Keep to a really healthy diet, including plenty of organic fruit and vegetables like carrots, lettuce, alfalfa sprouts and beetroot (*see* **General Heath Hints**).

Supplements

TH207 is a nutritional supplement especially made to support the thyroid (contains calcium, magnesium, Siberian Ginseng, niacinamide (B3), liquorice root, vitamin A, L-glutamine and amino acids). This is not a cure for thyroid problems, but this supplement aids thyroid functioning.

235

Also take a 1g linseed oil capsule for essential fats. A good multi-vitamin/mineral. ● [BC]

A vital nutrient for an underactive thyroid is iodine. Kombu seaweed, found in major health stores, is rich in iodine; or take a daily kelp supplement. Other supplements known to help an underactive thyroid are zinc citrate, selenium and the amino acid L-Tyrosine. As supplements for this condition tend to be very specialized, see a qualified nutritionist who can devise a programme for your specific body needs.

For an overactive thyroid, take a B complex daily to support the nerves and combat the effects of stress.

A thyroid supplement containing natural thyroxine called Armour Thyroid is available with a prescription. For further details, call 01435 882880.

Reading
Thyroid Problems by Patsy Westcott, £5.99, Thorsons.
The Riddle of Illness by Stephen E Langer MD, £10.99, Keats.

Hints
Many readers have found that taking stabilized aloe vera juice has helped their overall health when suffering thyroid problems. If you have thyroid problems it would be wise to consult a doctor who is also a qualified nutritionist (*see* **Useful Information** *for further details*). Smoking is known to make an underactive thyroid worse – so give up smoking.

Other readers have found that their thyroid function normalized after treatment from a homeopath. Others who are taking a natural progesterone supplement instead of HRT have also seen improvements (*see* **Menopause** *for details of natural progesterone*).

TINNITUS

Sufferers of tinnitus experience a constant noise or ringing sound in one or both ears. The condition can have a variety of causes which include exposure to loud noise, compacted wax, spinal misalignment, food sensitivities and poor circulation to the ears. Beta-blockers and aspirin can lead to tinnitus as a long-term side-effect.

Diet

Avoiding cows' milk, yeast, sugar and saturated fats may help (*see* **Allergies** *and* **Catarrh** *and* **General Health Hints**).

Supplements

Muccolyte containing vitamin C, potassium and hesperdin to clear sinuses. GLA, an essential fatty acid and 200iu of vitamin E to help circulation. Plus 30mg of zinc citrate for two months as tinnitus is often associated with a deficiency in zinc. Garlic, taken with main meals, helps to cleanse the sinuses and ginkgo biloba is known to improve micro circulation. • **[NC]**

Reading

Self-Help For Tinnitus by Arthur White, £2.99, Thorsons.

Hints

Have your teeth and gums checked as impacted wisdom teeth and tooth decay can cause this problem. When we grind our teeth over many years the jaw can be misaligned, this is known as TMJ (Temporo–Mandibular Joint Syndrome). Dentists who specialize in treating TMJ problems can make a small brace to be worn at night which helps to hold the jaw in its correct position, which often alleviates tinnitus (*for further details see* **Useful Information**). There is now a craniofacial pain clinic in London which is dedicated exclusively to the treatment of head, neck and facial pain; call 0171 637 5797 for further details.

Cranial osteopathy or chiropractic can release built-up tensions in the head and neck which often cause tinnitus. Acupuncture has proved very beneficial to some sufferers (*see* **Useful Information** *for further details*).

Many readers report that after listening to sound therapy tapes their tinnitus is much improved. For details and a brochure contact: Samonas UK, PO Box 1, Stibbard, Fakenham, Norfolk NR21 OES. Tel: 0956 701059.

Tinnitus helpline for up-to-date research on 0345 090210, 10am–3pm, Monday to Friday.

TONGUE PROBLEMS

Traditional Chinese doctors see the state of the tongue as an indicator of the patient's overall condition. A healthy tongue should be moist and clean, with little or no coating. Dryness of the tongue is usually an indication of dehydration. The tongue is usually coated in people with poor oral hygiene or those who smoke excessively. A coating on the tongue can also be linked to poor digestion and toxicity in the body. It can also suggest a sluggish liver, which again is related to the digestive system. Candida can produce a thick white coating on the tongue in severe cases (*see* **Candida**).

Diet

Avoid sugar-based and any junk and pre-packaged foods which are high in salt and sugar. Eat plenty of fresh green vegetables that have been lightly steamed to retain their vitamin content. Avoid red meat which can putrefy in the gut. Drink at least six glasses of filtered water daily to help remove toxins (*see* **General Health Hints**).

Supplements

Take a course of acidophilus which helps to replace the good bacteria in the intestinal tract and aids digestion. Also take a digestive enzyme with main meals to help break down the food and improve absorption of nutrients. • **[NC]**

The herb milk thistle is an excellent liver cleanser. • **[BLK]**

If you follow this regime, the problems with your digestive and elimination systems often clear completely (*see also* **Constipation** *and* **General Health Hints**).

Reading

Food Combining in 30 Days by Kathryn Marsden, £4.99, Thorsons.

TONGUE PROBLEMS – Geographical Tongue

This condition is so-called because the tongue often resembles a map, with discoloration of the tongue forming irregular shapes on the tongue's surface. Usually it disappears of its own accord, but sensitivity to certain foods can exacerbate the condition. See a kinesiologist who can determine if you have a specific allergy which could aggravate the tongue.

Diet

Avoid all spicy foods, vinegar and alcohol as they particularly irritate the membranes of the mouth. Eat plenty of silica-rich foods such as fresh vegetables and fruit (*see* **General Health Hints**).

Supplements

CT241 made from a blend of herbs and plant enzymes that provide nutrients involved in the formation of connective tissue such as kelp, vitamin C, manganese, silica, horsetail, boron and digestive enzymes to improve absorption of nutrients from food. Take one with every meal. • **[BC]**

Take friendly bacteria like acidophilus daily for one month plus a good multi-vitamin/mineral, as well as B vitamins every day.

Hints
Tea tree oil, a natural antiseptic, can be used as a mouthwash. Some sufferers report an improvement after taking a garlic capsule before breakfast every day.

TRAVEL SICKNESS
Stress, anxiety, a stuffy environment or too much food prior to travel can often make symptoms worse. If you are travelling by car or coach do not read while the vehicle is moving and look towards the horizon, which helps to stabilize the balancing mechanisms in the inner ear.

Diet
Eat light meals before travel and avoid oily or fatty foods which are hard to digest. Eat small amounts of fruit or rice cakes.

Supplements
Ginger is very effective in preventing nausea and travel sickness; take ginger capsules two hours before travelling and again, half an hour before you leave. If you are on a long trip, take a ginger capsule every hour on the road. The stress created by apprehension about travel sickness can compound the symptoms. To help prevent this, try a magnesium compound every hour before travelling. • **[BLK]**

Hints

Acupressure can help to control motion sickness. See a reflexologist who will show you which points to treat, or wear Sea Bands, which work on a similar principle; available from most chemists. Homeopathy is excellent for travel sickness – try homeopathic *petrol* or ask at your local pharmacy for a treatment to match your specific symptoms.

TREMORS

Tremors may have many different causes including excessive consumption of alcohol or caffeine, anxiety, an overactive thyroid gland and Parkinson's Disease. Occasionally tremors may be inherited. This can make it difficult to treat, though certain supplements may reduce the extent of the problem.

Diet

Avoid any strong stimulants like alcohol, spicy foods, cola type drinks, strong tea, coffee and chocolate (*see* **General Health Hints**).

Supplements

GLA, an essential fatty acid taken twice daily, helps repair nerve endings. Magnesium 400mg and calcium 200mg work together in the body to stabilize the nervous system.

Try Executive B formula which contains herbs like valerian root and passion flower, together with B vitamins and magnesium for the nervous system. • **[BLK]**

Hints

Some readers have found relief by plunging the affected limb into cold water for a few minutes each day. Acupuncture has also helped many people (*see* **Useful**

Information *for further details*).

VARICOSE VEINS

Varicose veins are distorted and dilated veins usually found in the legs. Anything which slows the return of blood from the leg to the heart will aggravate this condition. Development of varicose veins is closely linked with constipation, so avoid excessive straining which causes blood to flow into the lower half of the body. Being overweight doesn't help. Avoid crossing your legs which impedes blood flow from the legs. Many women develop varicose veins during pregnancy because the pregnant womb can obstruct blood flow from the veins. There is some hereditary component with varicose veins, as they do tend to run in families. If anyone has varicose veins in your family, bear in mind that prevention is more effective than treating them later.

Diet
Include plenty of fruit and vegetables in your diet, especially apricots, blackberries, cherries, rosehips and buckwheat, all of which contain rutin, a natural remedy for improving elasticity of veins. Avoid all junk foods that contain sugar and salt, as well as strong tea and coffee. Also avoid all foods that take a long time to pass through the bowel like red meat and refined foods such as cakes, biscuits and white bread. Organic raw linseeds are excellent for bowel cleansing. Initially, take a dessertspoon daily; gradually increase to one tablespoon. Drink at least six glasses of water every day. Aloe vera juice daily in fresh vegetable or fruit juice (*see* **General Health Hints**).

Supplements
Silica is an excellent mineral for toughening up veins; try

Silica Compound daily for at least three months. Gingko biloba is well known for improving circulation, but make sure it is a full strength capsule. Take 2g of vitamin C with bioflavonoids, along with 500iu of vitamin E daily, to help strengthen veins and improve blood flow. • [BLK]

The herb butcher's broom has proved successful in helping varicose veins and haemorrhoids. By taking 500–1,000mg each day you should see an improvement in the circulation in the lower limbs. This herb can also have a laxative effect. Witch hazel extracted from the plant can be taken in capsule form as it is full of flavonoids which increases resistance in capillaries. • [S]

Hints

Get plenty of fresh air and walk for at least 30 minutes every day. If you are fit enough take aerobic exercise, skipping, dancing, swimming or rebounding. Apply a little vitamin E cream mixed with two drops of juniper oil topically where the skin is sore.

Use cold compresses to reduce swelling. Many readers have found relief through acupuncture, wearing support tights and putting their feet and legs up against a wall for at least ten minutes daily to give the legs a total rest. I suffered from varicose veins after working as an air stewardess for nearly ten years, which meant that I was standing for many hours at a stretch. After having the veins removed, this has led to continually cold feet. Heed my warning if veins run in your family or if you have a job which requires long hours on your feet: make sure you put your feet up when you can and wear support tights. This will pay dividends in later life. As already mentioned, avoid constipation at all costs.

VEGETARIANISM

Vegetarianism is gaining popularity in Britain as the benefits of a vegetarian diet become clear and the potential hazards of eating meat (the BSE crisis is a case in point) emerge. Vegetarians enjoy better health than meat eaters, are less likely to be admitted to hospital and have a reduced risk of major killers like heart disease and cancer. However, vegetarians can sometimes have an unhealthy diet because they may eat a lot of dairy products, particularly cheese, to make up for the fact that they are not eating meat. Dairy products are generally high in saturated fat and are very high on the list of problem foods as far as food intolerance is concerned. Some people believe that if they do not eat dairy products they may become deficient in calcium. However, there is some evidence to suggest that we have great difficulty in absorbing calcium from dairy products once the milk has been pasteurized.

Diet

Green leafy vegetables, raw sesame seeds and fish are good sources of calcium. Any restricted diet may bring with it potential deficiencies. Vegetarians are at increased risk of B12 and iron deficiency compared to meat eaters, but this is only a problem in vegans who eat no animal produce as B12 is found in dairy products. The diet should be high in wholemeal bread, pasta, oat-based cereals, beans and pulses, brown rice, soya bean curd, vegetables and fruit. Wheat germ is packed with vitamin B and can be sprinkled onto cereals and soups.

Supplements

If you are anaemic, take a tonic like Spatone which includes vitamin C and B needed for iron absorption. From all good health stores (*see under* **Anaemia**).

Take a vegetarian multi-vitamin/mineral tablet which is high in zinc, iron and folic acid. • **[BC]**

244

Reading
The Teenage Vegetarian Survival Guide by Grose and Jones, £3.50, Red Fox. To order, call 0171 436 5122.
Vegan Nutrition: Pure & Simple by Michael Klapper, £7.50, Vegan Society. To order call 0181 877 9993.

VERRUCAS

Verrucas are warts that occur on the soles of the feet. They are caused by a virus and can be passed from person to person. This condition is usually a sign that your immune system is at a low ebb.

Diet
Keep your diet full of foods that contain immune-boosting nutrients such as fruits and vegetables, and wholegrains. Avoid foods that tend to depress immune function such as sugar and products made with refined white flour (*see* **Exhaustion** *and* **General Health Hints**).

Supplements
2g of vitamin C, which is anti-viral. The herb echinacea boosts the immune system and golden seal is anti-viral. A good anti-oxidant formula every day for six months. • **[BLK]**

Hints
Rub a crushed garlic clove twice a day into the affected area. Vitamin E and A oils have also been successful in the removal of verrucas – pierce a capsule of the oil and apply to the affected area. Chinese herbal medicine and homeopathy have proved helpful (*see* **Useful Information** *for details*). You could also tape a small piece of banana skin with the inside surface in contact with the verruca, change daily. There is an enzyme in the banana skin

which attacks the verruca. Many readers have written to say that, although somewhat bizarre, this remedy really does work!

VERTIGO

Vertigo is a term used to describe a sensation of dizziness and loss of balance, sometimes accompanied by nausea. It can be caused by impacted earwax, blockage of the eustation tube or by viral infections of the balancing mechanism in the inner ear. Vertigo can also be caused by high blood pressure or too much catarrh (*see* **Catarrh**). Dizziness can also be a sign of iron deficiency (*see* **Anaemia**), or low blood sugar (*see* **Low Blood Sugar**), or low blood pressure (*see also* **Low Blood Pressure**).

Diet
Cut out cows' milk and cheese from your diet for one month. Replace them with rice milk, which is non-dairy. Avoid all saturated fats and do not fry food. Eat plenty of fresh vegetables, fruits, brown rice, brown bread and fresh garlic. A food combining diet can be helpful (*see* **General Health Hints**).

Supplements
Garlic is very cleansing if taken regularly. Ginger capsules to aid the feeling of nausea and dizziness. The herb gingko biloba, 60–120mg of standardized extract daily to improve circulation in the head. 2g of vitamin C plus a multivitamin/mineral. • **[FSC]**

Hints
See a chiropractor or cranial osteopath to make sure your neck and spine are not misaligned as this can cause

problems in the ear. Hypnotherapy and acupuncture have helped in some cases (*see* **Useful Information** *for further details*). Many readers report that after listening to sound therapy tapes their vertigo is much improved. For details and a brochure contact: Samonas UK, PO Box 1, Stibbard, Fakenham, Norfolk NR 21 OES. Tel: 0956 701059.

High blood pressure and beta blockers have been known to cause vertigo in some people. Therefore, if you have been taking prescription drugs for a long period of time, check with your GP.

VIRAL INFECTIONS
Viral infections can manifest themselves in many ways in the body, but by far the most common examples are colds and flu. Our susceptibility to viral infections and how badly we are affected by them depends on the strength of the strain of the virus and how healthy our immune system is. Keeping our immune system healthy is essential to preventing and combating viral infections. Viruses can sometimes be very difficult to shake off and may leave the body weakened for some time. Chronic fatigue syndrome is thought in many sufferers to be due at least in part to a viral infection.

Diet
Avoid sugar which can compromise the strength of the immune system and worsen any existing viral infection. Eat a diet rich in fresh fruits and vegetables that are high in vitamin C, which is known to be a potent anti-viral agent (*see* **General Health Hints**).

Supplements
Echinacea is a natural immune booster; try a high potency

like Blackmores Echinacea ACE + zinc for at least two months.

The herb golden seal is anti-viral; take a combination supplement like golden seal, echinacea and cat's claw. Three capsules daily for six weeks. Grapefruit seed extract is anti-viral and anti-bacterial. • **[S]**

Reading
All Day Energy by Kathryn Marsden, £4.99, Thorsons.
Boost Your Immune System by Jennifer Meek, £5.95, ION Press.

Hints
People who suffer regularly from viral infections are often lacking in essential fats (*see* **Fats You Need to Eat**).

Ongoing headaches from post-viral syndrome can often be alleviated by cranial osteopathy (*see* **Useful Information** *for further details*).

VITILIGO

Vitiligo is a condition which causes patches of skin to lose their pigmentation. The darker the natural skin colour, the more obvious the condition is. The causes of vitiligo are not known, but it is very likely that the immune system is involved and has been linked to low stomach acid, a malfunctioning thyroid and vitamin B deficiency.

Supplements
Betaine hydrochloride – research has shown that most sufferers of vitiligo have a lack of hydrochloric acid (HCl) in their stomachs. Supplementation with HCl at meal times in the form of betaine hydrochloride may be helpful in correcting this disorder over a period of months. HCl

supplements should not be used by those with a history of ulcers of the digestive tract without the advice of a qualified health practitioner. It should only be used with main meals and if any excessive warmth or irritation is experienced in the stomach after using, the dosage should be reduced at the next meal to a level where this does not occur.

Deficiencies in various B vitamins especially B5, B6 and PABA are also linked to vitiligo as they are needed for proper HCl activity and others are required for normal pigmentation. Take a potent B complex regularly.

Zinc deficiencies are a common factor in those with a lack of stomach acid. Zinc supplementation of 15–45mg may help restore digestive activity in the stomach and is also one of the most important nutrients for general skin health. • **[FSC]**

Also take a multi-vitamin/mineral daily. Essential fatty acids stimulate hormone function and help to feed the skin (*see* **Fats You Need to Eat**).

WARTS

Warts are caused by a virus and will often disappear of their own accord. Persistent warts can be a sign of a weakened immune system (*see* **Viral Infections**).

Diet

Keep your diet full of foods that contain immune system boosting nutrients such as fruits and vegetables, and wholegrains. Avoid foods that tend to depress immune function such as sugar (*see* **General Health Hints**).

Supplements

Rub liquid garlic, mixed with a little vitamin C cream, twice daily into the wart; also eat raw garlic or take a garlic capsule. Vitamins E and A have also been successful in the removal of warts – pierce a capsule and apply the contents directly to the affected area. It is also important to boost the immune system; take a good anti-oxidant formula that contains vitamins C, E, A, beta carotene and the minerals zinc and selenium.

Hints
Chinese herbal medicine and homeopathy have proved very successful in the removal of warts (*see* **Useful Information** *for further details*). Many readers have used apple cider vinegar on a plaster over the wart. By changing regularly and adding more vinegar, the warts have disappeared after 2 weeks.

WATER ON THE KNEE
Water on the knee is caused by inflammation of the fluid-filled sack that surrounds the knee joint. This condition is most commonly caused by injury to the knee or some arthritic process (*see under* **Arthritis**).

Diet
Reduce all acid-forming foods in your diet like meat, full cream milk, cheese and chocolate. Avoid junk foods and white bread and cakes, which are not only acid-forming but high in salt, which can aggravate water retention. Eat plenty of foods high in potassium – bananas, nuts and seeds, along with organic vegetables like cabbage and broccoli. Include oily fish in your diet (*see* **General Health Hints**).

Supplements
Try using a natural herbal diuretic made from dandelion leaves which helps to reduce swelling. Take chloride

compound to lessen inflammation, plus 1g of vitamin C with bioflavonoids, plus bilberry extract and silica to help repair and strengthen tissues. • **[BLK]**

The pineapple extract bromelain is highly anti-inflammatory and, when symptoms are particularly severe, take 500–1,000mg a day on an empty stomach. • **[FSC]**

Hints
Perseverance with this regime is important as knee problems can take some time to heal. Acupuncture and homeopathy have proved very helpful to many sufferers (*see* **Useful Information** *for further details*).

WATER RETENTION – Oedema
Fluid retention is most commonly seen in the hands, feet and around the eyes. It is a very common symptom which can be caused by hormone imbalance, the Pill, orthodox HRT and food sensitivities. Very occasionally fluid retention may be due to a serious problem affecting the heart, liver or kidneys.

Diet
Avoid all junk, pre-packaged and sugar-based foods, especially those that contain sodium (salt). Cut down on tea, coffee, colas and salty foods like crisps. Eat a healthy diet of fresh vegetables, fruits and whole grains like brown rice, barley, oat-based cereals and brown bread and pasta. Drink at least one litre of bottled or filtered water every day (*see* **General Health Hints**).

Supplements
Celery seed extract plus 1g of potassium ascorbate, a form of vitamin C which helps fluid drainage. A multi-vitamin for

women like Femforte. Take a B complex and 50–100mg of B6 for three weeks as B6 is a natural diuretic. Junipearas, a homeopathic product to remove excess body water. • **[NC]**

Hints
Dandelion tea is a natural diuretic and a good source of potassium. Regular exercise like walking or swimming helps this condition.

WEIGHT PROBLEMS

I receive so many sad letters from people who are desperate to lose weight. The answer is definitely not to starve yourselves or to keep trying out fad diets. The conventional medical establishment still see the only cause of being overweight as over-eating and continue to advocate the calorie approach to weight loss which is almost never effective in the long term. Repeated dieting can reduce the rate at which your body is able to burn food for energy (the metabolic rate). So, over a number of years it becomes more and more difficult to lose weight, even though you may be practically starving yourself from time to time. Also, dieting can reduce the level of sugar in the blood and the level of certain chemicals in the brain which can lead to binge eating and mood changes. Allergies to certain foods cause fluid retention which add to the weight problem (*see* **Allergies**). Generally speaking, repeated dieting only reduces the nutritional value of the diet still further, leading to deficiencies that may have an important impact on health in the long term.

Diet
The secret to losing weight is not to diet, but to work healthy eating into your daily life. First of all, make sure you eat

regularly during the day. Regular meals will help keep your metabolic rate normalized while also helping to maintain your blood sugar level and so prevent bingeing. Keep your diet based around whole, unprocessed and unadulterated foods such as fresh fruits and vegetables, wholemeal bread, brown rice, barley and wholewheat pasta. Wherever possible, avoid unnecessary saturated fat found in red meat and dairy products. Drink plenty of filtered or bottled water which helps speed the elimination of toxins from the body. Common food allergens are wheat and dairy produce made from cows' milk. Avoid these for a month and see if your weight drops. Try rice milk and eat soda bread, oat and rice cakes.

Many people say that food combining has helped them to lose weight on a permanent basis. The principle is not to eat protein (eg meat, fish, cheese, eggs), with starch (eg bread, potatoes, rice, pasta) at the same meal. Either proteins *or* starch are mixed with neutral foods (vegetables other than the potato) at each meal. Food combining works by allowing more complete digestion of food (*see* **General Health Hints**).

Supplements
Take a good quality multi-vitamin and mineral tablet every day and make sure you take one tablespoon of essential fatty acids in an oil formula every day (*for details, see* **Fats You Need to Eat**). Chromium Picolinate helps to reduce sugar cravings. Take two drops in water daily for at least six weeks. • **[NC]**

There is a supplement extracted from an Asian fruit called garcinia cambogia which contains hydroxycitric acid (HCA). In many tests it has shown an ability to curb appetite, reduce food intake by 10% and regulate production of fats and cholesterol. One of the most potent brands is CitriMax Forte, which also includes manganese ascorbate and chromium to assist blood sugar levels, which helps prevent sugar cravings. It should be taken 30 minutes before each meal as part of a healthy diet. It may take a few weeks to see results, but this is a safer way to lose weight. **(Not to be taken if pregnant or anorexic.)** For further details, call either 0171 436 5122 or 0121 433 3727.

Reading

Weight Control by Stephen Terrass, £4.99, Thorsons.
The Fat Burner Diet by Patrick Holford, £5.99 ION Press. To order, call 0181 877 9993.
Food Combining in 30 Days by Kathryn Marsden, £4.99, Thorsons.

Hints

Dandelion tea or pure root dandelion coffee are great for cleansing the liver and in studies have shown to help weight loss. Often women on a low calorie intake tend to become malnourished and, when encouraged to eat healthy food more frequently, they actually lose weight. Eat as much healthy food as you like, which tends to stimulate the metabolism, thereby improving overall health and weight loss. Regular exercise is vital not only for losing weight but for overall health. Try and exercise for at least 30 minutes every day.

Oestrogen can cause weight gain and water retention if your body is low in progesterone. If you think you have a hormone imbalance and would like a free progesterone and Food Allergy Factsheet, send an SAE to: Higher Nature Ltd, The Nutrition Centre, Burwash Common, East Sussex TN19 7LX. For further information on natural progesterone, send £2 to: The Natural Progesterone Information Service, BCM 4315, London WC1N 3XX.

If you suffer from eating disorders and need help, send a large SAE to: The Eating Disorders Association, Sackville Place, 44 Magdalen St, Norwich NR3 1JU or call their helpline 01603 621414, open Monday–Friday, 9.30am–6pm or their youth helpline 01603 765050, open Monday–Friday, 4pm–6pm. A membership scheme is available. Or try reading *Anorexia & Bulimia* by Julia Buckroyd, £4.99, Element Books.

Well, here we are at the end of the hints section. We realize that we could go on and on without end, but John and I have tried to give you a good base from which to find more help for your specific condition. I am sorry that I am too busy to answer individual health queries any longer, but if you read through the Index of Useful Information and Addresses, you will find associations that offer more in-depth help. I am always keen to learn and love to hear from practitioners, doctors or the public if you find something that has helped a specific condition, so that I can pass this information on, hopefully to help others. I can be reached via my publishers. Good luck and good health.

Hazel Courteney and Dr John Briffa

Index of Useful Information and Addresses

ACUPUNCTURE
Practitioners use fine, sterile needles inserted into specific points to regulate energy flow and restore health.

To find your nearest practitioner, send an SAE to: British Acupuncture Council Park House, 206–208 Latimer Road, London W10 6RE.

ALEXANDER TECHNIQUE
Teaches you how to use your body more efficiently and how to have balance and poise with minimum tension in order to avoid pain, strain and injury.

To find your nearest practitioner, send an SAE to: The Society of Teachers of Alexander Technique, 20 London House, 266 Fulham Road, London SW10 9EL. Tel: 0171 351 0828.

ALOE VERA CENTRE
If you have any problems finding good quality aloe vera juice or would like further information on the healing properties of aloe vera, send a large SAE to: The Aloe Vera Centre, Gardiner House, 3/9 Broomhill Road, London SW18 4JQ. Tel: 0181 871 5083/5205.

AROMATHERAPY
The use of essential oils to improve health and well-being, by massage, inhalation, compresses and baths. Excellent for

reducing stress and anxiety.

For a register of practitioners, send an SAE with a cheque/postal order for £2 to: International Federation of Aromatherapists, Stamford House, 2–4 Chiswick High Road, London W4 1TH. Tel: 0181 742 2605.

Or send an SAE to: International Society of Professional Aromatherapists, 82 Ashby Road, Hinckley, Leicestershire LE10 1SN.

AUSTRALIAN BUSH FLOWER ESSENCES

Traditionally flower essences have been used to heal emotions and act as a catalyst for healing, they work on subtle energies of our bodies and help to unblock emotional or personality problems. Specific flower essences are available to suit your particular condition from Serena Smith who is a holistic therapist and healer. If you would like to receive a brochure or further information on flower essences, please send an SAE to: PO Box 3896, London NW3 7DS or call 0171 431 6153.

BACH FLOWER THERAPY

A healing system used to treat emotional problems such as fear and hopelessness. The liquid remedies are made from the flowers of wild plants, bushes and trees.

To find your nearest practitioner, send an SAE to: The Bach Centre, Mount Vernon, Sotwell, Wallingford, Oxfordshire OX10 0PX. Tel: 01491 834678.

BIO-CRANIAL OSTEOPATHY

A gentle method of osteopathy concentrating on nerves in the head, neck and shoulders. Many readers have reported success with ME (Chronic Fatigue Syndrome) and arthritis from this therapy.

To find your nearest practitioner, send an SAE to: The International Bio-Cranial Academy, PO Box 44, Bangor, County Down BT20 3SY. Tel: 01247 270626.

CHINESE HERBAL MEDICINE

The concept of restoring an uninterrupted flow of chi, the vital energy of the body. Be aware that if you are taking large doses of herbs they are extremely potent and you may want to have a liver function test at regular intervals during your treatment.

For a register of practitioners, send a large SAE and cheque/postal order for £1.50 to: Register of Chinese Herbal Medicine, PO Box 400, Wembley, Middlesex HA9 9NZ.

CHIROPRACTIC

Gentle manipulation to treat disorders of the joints and muscles and their effect on the nervous system. Chiropractors treat the entire body to bring it back into balance and restore health. I personally prefer being gently manipulated by a chiropractor to osteopathy which can be a little more radical.

For a register of practitioners, send a large SAE and a cheque/postal order for £2 to: The British Chiropractic Association, Equity House, 29 Whitley Street, Reading, Berkshire RG2 0EG. Tel: 01734 757557.

Or send an SAE to: McTimmony Chiropractic Association, 21 High Street, Eynsham, Oxfordshire OX8 1HE. Tel: 01865 880974.

COLONIC HYDROTHERAPY

Method of cleansing the colon to gently flush away toxic waste, gas, accumulated faeces and mucus deposits. Check with your GP before undertaking this therapy. Colonics are very useful if you are chronically constipated or have taken antibiotics or painkillers which can cause constipation.

To find your nearest practitioner, send an SAE to: Colonic International Association, 16 Englands Lane, London NW3 4TG. Tel/Fax: 0171 483 1595.

COLOUR THERAPY

There is plenty of evidence to show that colour does affect our mood and behaviour, as different colours emit an aura of their own which our bodies absorb.

To find your nearest practitioner, send an SAE to: International Association of Colour Therapy, 137 Hendon Lane, Finchley, London N3 3PR.

COUNSELLING

If you, or a member of your family, is in need of professional counselling, send an SAE to: British Association for Counselling (BAC), 1 Regent Place, Rugby CV21 2PJ. Tel: 01788 578328.

CRANIAL OSTEOPATHY

Therapists use hands to release resistance in tissues, bones and fluids, often resulting in revitalization of the system. Many readers report benefits from such conditions as facial pain, migraine, chronic fatigue and even arthritis after having a few treatments which release nerves, thus restoring natural energy flow.

To find your nearest practitioner, send an SAE to: Cranial Osteopathic Association, 478 Baker Street, Enfield, Middlesex EN1 3QS. Tel: 0181 367 5561.

CRYSTAL THERAPY

Crystals can both receive and transmit signals or energy. A good healer generates healing energy into a crystal which is then transferred to the patient. The crystal can then be used for healing purposes without the need for the healer to be present.

To find your nearest practitioner, send an SAE to: Affiliation of Crystal Healing Organisations, 46 Lower Green Road, Esher, Surrey KT10 8HD. Tel: 0181 398 7252.

GENERAL ORGANIZATIONS

If you want to know more about specific alternative therapies, the following organizations will be happy to give you advice and put you in touch with the practitioners and societies that now meet with their high standards of practice and therapy.

British Complementary Medicine Association, 39 Prestbury Road, Cheltenham, Gloucestershire GL52 2PT. Tel: 01242 226770

Council for Complementary and Alternative Medicine, Park House, 206–208 Latimer Road, London W10 6RE. Tel: 0181 968 3862.

Institute for Complementary Medicine, PO Box 194, London SE16 1QZ. Tel: 0171 237 5165.

HALE CLINIC

This clinic is the largest alternative treatment centre in Europe with over 100 practitioners, many of whom are also qualified medical doctors.

The Hale Clinic, 7 Park Crescent, London W1N 3HE. Tel: 0171 631 0156.

HEALING

The healer is a channel for the transfer of healing energy to the patient.

To find your nearest practitioner, send an SAE to: National Federation of Spiritual Healers, Old Manor Farm Studio, Church Street, Sunbury-on-Thames, Middlesex TW16 6RG. Tel: 0891 616080 (Monday to Friday, 9am–5pm).

I know there are hundreds of very able healers in the UK, but I would like to mention four from whom I have personally benefitted. Dennis Sinclair specializes in bone problems; he can be contacted on 0181 902 0931. David Cunningham, who works all over the UK, can be contacted on 01932 846 345 or 0973 638910, or in Ireland on 00 353 283 3538. Seka Nikolic and her brother Momo Kovacevic have extraordinary healing powers and specialize in helping people with ME (Chronic Fatigue Syndrome). At the time of going to press, they both work from the Hale Clinic in London. Tel: 0171 631 0156.

HEALTHRIGHT HEALTH REPORT

HealthRight is a service run by two medically qualified doctors who also specialize in nutrition and vitamin advice. They will send you a full report on your current state of health with recommendations on any necessary improvements you could make, including dietary and lifestyle advice for £14.95. For further information and to obtain a HealthRight questionnaire for assessment, write to HealthRight, 1 Pawnshop Passage, Lough, Lincolnshire LN11 9JQ or call 01507 600229.

HERBALISM

The practice of using plants to treat disease. Treatment may be given in the form of fluid extracts, tinctures, tablets and teas.

For a register of practitioners, send a large SAE with two first class stamps to: National Institute of Medical Herbalists, 56 Longbrook Street, Exeter, Devon EX4 6AH. Tel: 01392 426022.

Potter's make one of the most comprehensive ranges of herbs available in the UK and for further details of their remedies and a stockist near you, call Potter's Herbal Products on 01942 234761.

HOMEOPATHY

Homeopaths prescribe remedies in the form of tablets, granules, powders or liquids, which are thought to stimulate the body's healing processes.

To find your nearest practitioner, send an SAE to: Society of Homeopaths, 2 Artizan Road, Northampton NN1 4HU. Tel: 01604 21400.

Or send an SAE to: The UK Homeopathic Medical

Association, 6 Livingstone Road, Gravesend, Kent DA12 5DZ. Tel: 01474 560336.

To find a doctor who is also a homeopath, send an A4 SAE with three x first class stamps to: Homeopathic Trust, 2 Powis Place, Great Ormond Street, London WC1N 3HT.

HYPNOTHERAPY
By allowing external distractions to fade, the therapy allows you to fully relax and understand the root cause of many of your problems, phobias and addictions.

To find your nearest practitioner, send an SAE to: National Council of Psychotherapists and Hypnotherapy Register, 24 Rickmondsworth Road, Watford, Hertfordshire WD1 7HT. Tel : 01590 644913

INSTITUTE OF OPTIMUM NUTRITION
The Institute of Optimum Nutrition print a wonderful quarterly booklet which costs £1.95 a quarter, plus p&p. This booklet is packed with up-to-date health news and the latest research in alternative medicine, which I often refer to when I need up to the minute information. The Institute also holds seminars on health and have in-house nutritionists. ION also have an excellent alternative health library and database. For details, contact the Institute of Optimum Nutrition, Blades Court, Deodar Road, London SW15 2NU. Tel: 0181 877 9993. Monday to Friday, 10am–5pm.

IRIDOLOGY
A method of analysis rather than treatment, based on the theory that the whole body is reflected in the eyes. Using a magnifier, the practitioner examines the visible parts of the eyes to pinpoint physical weaknesses or potential areas of trouble.

To find your nearest practitioner, send an SAE to: International Association of Clinical Iridologists, 853 Finchley Road, London NW1 8LX.

KINESIOLOGY

Science of testing muscle response to discover areas of impaired energy and function in the body. Kinesiology is especially useful if you think you have an allergic reaction either to a food or an external allergen.

To find your nearest practitioner, send an SAE to: The Association for Systematic Kinesiology, 39 Browns Road, Surbiton, Surrey KT5 8ST. Tel: 0181 399 3215.

MAGNOTHERAPY

Regular doses of magnet therapy can help boost energy levels, improve circulation and accelerate healing. Many people have also found relief from wearing magnetized jewellery and using magnetized products for pain relief.

Magnet Therapy Centres:
The Hale Clinic, 7 Park Crescent, London W1N 3HE. Tel: 0171 631 0156.

Magnotherapy products are available from: Nikken UK, Unit 7, Landmere Lane, Edwalton, Nottingham NG12 4DE. Tel: 0115 9456595.

Acar-Sud, Westfield House, Hampton Court Road, East Molesey, Surrey KT8 9BX. Tel : 0181 977 1699.

MANUAL LYMPHATIC DRAINAGE

A very gentle pulsing massage which helps to drain the lymph nodes thereby reducing swelling and pain related to the lymph tissues.

To find your nearest practitioner, send an SAE to: MLD UK, PO Box 149, Wallingford, Oxfordshire OX10 7LD.

NATUROPATHY

Practitioner uses diet, osteopathy, water therapy along with various supplements to treat the root cause of any illness, thereby boosting the immune system and hopefully restoring perfect health.

For a register of practitioners, send a large SAE and cheque or postal order for £2.50 to: General Council and Register of Naturopaths, 2 Goswell Road, Street, Somerset BA16 0JG. Tel : 01458 840072.

NUTRI CENTRE, The
The Nutri Centre, located on the lower ground floor of the Hale Clinic at 7 Park Crescent London, is unique in being able to supply almost every alternative product currently available in the UK, including specialized practitioner products. The Nutri Centre offers an excellent and reliable mail order service for all its products. Tel: 0171 436 5122 Fax: 0171 436 5171.

NUTRITIONAL OILS
Savant Distribution Ltd distribute Dr Udo Erasmus' oil and other nutritional oils. For more information, contact them at 7 Wayland Croft, Adel, Leeds, LS16 8LA. Tel: 0113 230 1993.

NUTRITIONAL THERAPY
Health care system using individual diet and supplement programmes to enhance food absorption, correct nutritional deficiencies, combat allergies and reduce toxic overload.

Send a large SAE plus £1 for information and a list of practitioners to: Society for the Promotion of Nutritional Therapy, PO Box 47, Heathfield, East Sussex TN21 8ZX. Tel: 01435 867007.

NUTRITIONIST WHO IS ALSO A DOCTOR
You will need to be referred by your own GP who will be able to find the address of your nearest practitioner by contacting: The British Society for Allergy & Environmental Medicine P O Box 28, Totton, Southampton SO40 2LA.

ORGANIC PRODUCE
The Soil Association produce a directory listing the

suppliers of organic produce throughout the country. To obtain a copy, send £3 to the Soil Association, 86 Colston Street, Bristol BS1 5BB or for further information, call 0117 929 0661.

OSTEOPATHY
A system of healing that works on the physical structure of the body. Practitioners use manipulation massage and stretching techniques.

To find your nearest practitioner, send an SAE to: Osteopathic Information Service, PO Box 2074, Reading, Berkshire RG1 4YR. Tel: 01734 512051.

POLARITY THERAPY
A therapist will use bodywork, awareness skills, diet and polarity stretching exercises to help the body and mind heal itself naturally. A very relaxing re-balancing therapy useful for extreme stress and fatigue.

To find your nearest practitioner, send an SAE to: United Kingdom Polarity Therapy Association, Monomark House, 27 Old Gloucester Street, London WC1N 3XX. Tel: 01524 67009.

PUBLISHERS
Here is a list of the numbers of all major publishers used in this book if you would prefer to order by mail :

Bantam Books	01624 675137
Element Books	01747 851339
Green Library	0171 385 0012
ION Press	0181 877 9993
Optima Press	01621 819600
Thorsons	0141 772 2281
Waterstones bookstores	01225 448595

QIGONG
An extremely gentle form of exercise which helps people with impaired mobility like severe arthritis. Anyone can practise Qigong and no special clothes are needed. For your nearest class or teacher, send a SAE to : The Tse Qi Gong Centre, PO Box 116, Manchester M20 3YN. Tel: 0161 434 5289.

READING – my favourite books
If you have difficulty in finding any of the recommended books, the Nutri Centre have an extensive library of self-help books and would be happy to order for you, or give assistance on specific subjects on 0171 436 5122.

Day Dream Diet: The Inner Game of Dieting, by Julia Hastings, £8.99, Touchstone Publications, PO Box 54, Haslemere, Surrey GU27 2RW.

Julia has a fresh approach to weight loss and eating disorders and this book teaches you how to use mental picturing to change how you perceive your body.

Fats That Heal and Fats That Kill, Dr Udo Erasmus, £14.50, Alive Books. To order, call 0181 877 9993.

Dr Erasmus is a world authority on fats and this book is a must for any health practitioner or doctor who wants to know in-depth information and correct research about fats and oils.

The Fats We Need To Eat, Jeannette Ewin, £6.99, Thorsons.

An excellent book for anyone who wants to understand more about which fats and oils are healthy and which ones can kill. Easy to read and very informative.

Food Combining in 30 Days by Kathryn Marsden, £4.99, Thorsons.

Food combining is marvellous for anyone suffering digestive problems, irritable bowel, hiatus hernia or people who simply want to stay fit or lose weight.

Healing Through Nutrition by Dr Melvyn R Werbach,

£16.99, Thorsons. To order from The Nutri Centre on 0171 436 5122.

Dr Werbach is a world authority on healing through nutrition and supplements. This book is a must for all doctors who want to know more about scientific evidence and expanded explanations which have not been possible in this book.

Here's Health magazine £2.10

My favourite alternative health magazine. Packed with up-to-date alternative research and helpful articles and hints that can help you on your path towards health via alternative means. An absolute must every month.

Homeopathy – A Practical Guide to Everyday Health Care by Robin Hayfield, Virgin Publishing, £9.99. To order telephone 0181 968 7554.

I found this an extremely informative, easy to read book for anyone who would like to know more about homeopathy.

Mental Health & Illness by Patrick Holford, £7.95, ION Press.

Many of us do not realize that problems often associated with mental health, mood swings, memory loss and dementia can be cured once diet and supplements are in balance.

The New Super Nutrition by Dr Richard Passwater, £5.99, Pocket Books. To order call 0171 436 5122.

Once I started this book I could not put it down; brilliantly researched and highly informative with specific vitamin supplement information.

Optimum Nutrition by Patrick Holford, £5.99, ION Press.

Packed with up-to-date ideas on nutrition and supplements. Written by one of the UK's leading nutritionists.

Spontaneous Healing by Dr Andrew Weil £19.55, published by Knops. To order, call 0171 436 5122.

Dr Weil has spent a lifetime trying to understand how

through the power of the mind, natural therapies and orthodox medicine can heal the body. He includes dozens of case studies which show how the power of the mind and good nutritional therapies can work miracles. I found this book completely riveting.

Testimony of Light by Helen Graves, £5.95, The C W Daniel Company Ltd. Available to order from Watkins Books on 0171 836 2182.

A magical story written by a nun about life after death. Whether you believe in life after death or not, this book makes compulsive reading.

What Doctors Don't Tell You by Lynne McTaggart, £7.99, Thorsons

Lynne McTaggart is the Editor of the informative monthly newsletter 'What Doctors Don't Tell You' and in this book Lynne gives a great insight into the medical establishment and hopefully will prevent you becoming another medical statistic.

REFLEXOLOGY

Works on the principle that reflex points on the hands and feet correspond to every part of the body. By working with pressure on these points, blockages in the energy pathways are released and encouraged to heal. Ideal to boost circulation.

To find your nearest practitioner, send an SAE to: The Association of Reflexologists, 27 Old Gloucester Street, London WC1N 3XX. Tel: 0990 673320.

Or send an SAE to: The British Reflexology Association, Monks Orchard, Whitbourne, Worcestershire WR6 5RB. Tel: 01886 821207.

TMJ (Temporo–Mandibular Joint Syndrome)

Many people who suffer migraines and persistent headaches in fact grind their teeth, which causes the jaw to become misaligned. I had good teeth removed and considerable amounts of surgery on my gums, which turned out to be unnecessary – I simply had TMJ, but many dentists have no knowledge of this condition.

To find your nearest practitioner, send an SAE to: The Cranio Group, Wretham Lodge, Priory Road, Forest Row, East Sussex RH18 5HR.

WHAT DOCTORS DON'T TELL YOU

What Doctors Don't Tell You is a monthly newsletter packed with alternative health information; but more importantly, endless advice on the side-effects of drugs. Anyone who has to take large amounts of medication should subscribe to this newsletter. £24.95 for a one year subscription, back issues are £2.90 each. For details, write to *What Doctors Don't Tell You*, 4 Wallace Road, London N1 2PG. Tel: 0171 354 4592.

YOGA

The ancient principles of yoga are beneficial for helping anyone who is going through a stressful period in their life. It teaches relaxation and breathing techniques, together with gentle stretching exercises which help keep the 'whole' self fit and healthy. Especially useful for keeping the back and body supple throughout life.

To find your nearest class, send an A5 SAE to: The British Wheel of Yoga, 1 Hamilton Place, Boston Road, Sleaford, Lincolnshire NG34 7ES. Tel/Fax : 01529 306851.

ALPHABETICAL INDEX OF HELPFUL HEALTH HINTS